Beauty Basics & Beyond

101 Ways to Keep Your HAIR and SKIN Fabulous

ESSENCE
BOOKS

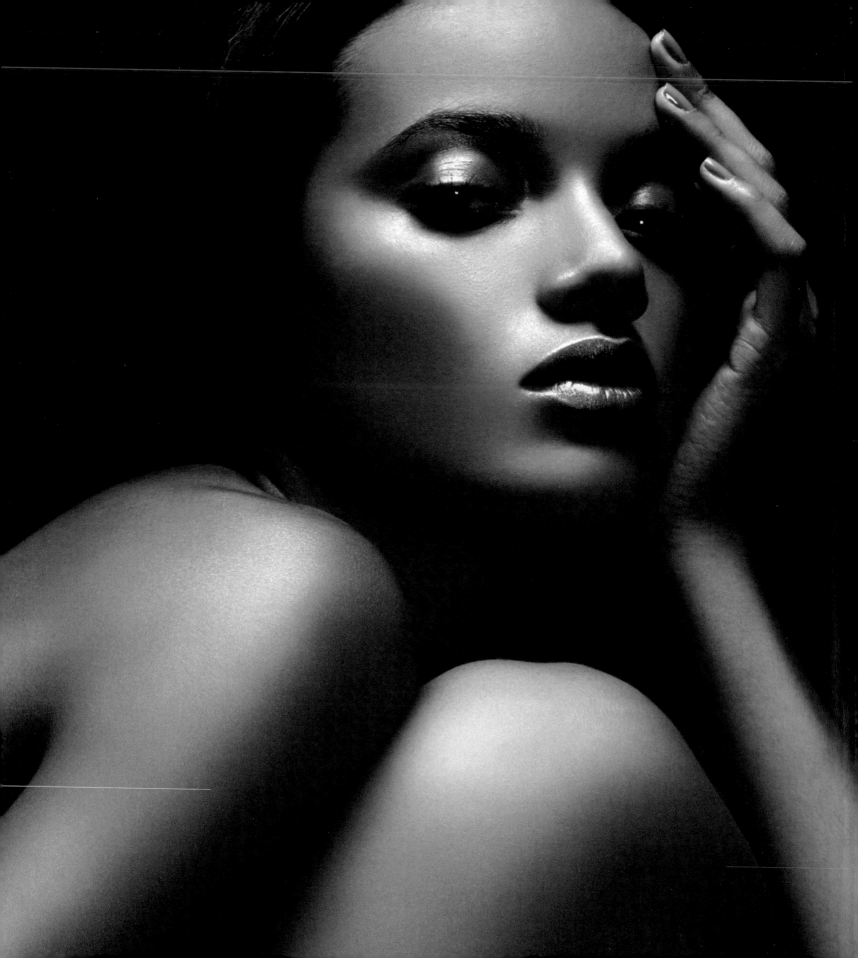

Beauty Basics & Beyond

101 Ways to Keep Your HAIR and SKIN Fabulous

Edited by Patricia Hinds
Introduction by Susan L. Taylor

ESSENCE BOOKS

Time Inc. Home Entertainment

Publisher: Richard Fraiman
Executive Director, Marketing Services: Carol Pittard
Director, Retail & Special Sales: Tom Mifsud
Marketing Director, Branded Businesses: Swati Rao
Director, New Product Development: Peter Harper
Assistant Financial Director: Steven Sandonato
Prepress Manager: Emily Rabin
Associate Book Production Manager: Suzanne Janso
Associate Prepress Manager: Anne-Michelle Gallero

Special thanks: Victoria Alfonso, Bozena Bannett, Alexandra Bliss, Glenn Buonocore, Bernadette Corbie, Robert Marasco, Brooke McGuire, Jonathan Polsky, Ilene Schreider, Adriana Tierno, Calandria Wells Britney Williams

Special thanks to Imaging: Patrick Dugan, Eddie Matros

ISBN: 1-932994-07-6
Library of Congress Control Number: 2005905673

We welcome your comments and suggestions about Essence Books. Please write to us at:
Essence Books
Attention: Book Editors
P.O. Box 11016
Des Moines, IA 50336-1016

If you would like to order any of our hardcover Collector's Edition books, please call us at (800) 327-6388. (Monday through Friday, 7:00 A.M.–8:00 P.M. or Saturday, 7:00 A.M.–6:00 P.M. Central Time)

Subscribe to Essence Magazine today! For fast service call (800) 274-9398 and mention code EEACN36.

Contributors

Editor-in-Chief: Patricia Hinds
Designer: Elizabeth Van Itallie
Writers: Julia Chance, Marcia Cole, Rozalynn Frazier, Jenyne Raines, Stephanie Scott
Editorial Assistants: Rehema Kahurananga, Nicole Sealey
Contributing Editors: Rosemarie Robotham, Linda Villarosa
Copy Editors: Nana Badu, Laura Larson
Beauty Consultants: John Atchison, Alfred Fornay, Deborah Simmons, M.D.
Interns: Lisa Acevedo, Stephanie Daye

Produced and packaged by Mignon Communications

Special thanks: Susan L. Taylor, Michelle Ebanks, Ed Lewis, Jan deChabert, Latoya Valmont, Fred Allen, Jean Borrie, Barbara Britton, Karen Brown, Vanessa Bush, Sherrill Clarke, Tom Colaprico, Michaela angela Davis, Pamela Edwards, Judy Jackson, Barbara Kelly, LaVon Leak-Wilks, Kathryn Leary, Sandra Martin, Cori M. Murray, Jonell Nash, Stephanie Stokes Oliver, Debra Parker, Constance Robotham-Reid, Leah Rudolfo, Cindy Schreibman, Akiba Solomon, Robin Stone, Mikki Taylor, Tasha Turner, Charlotte Wiggers

Special appreciation: Mark Anthony, Diane Bailey, Marvin Carrington, Djeneba Damba, Carla Gentry, Neeko, Mariam Sy

Acknowledgments: Marsha Augustin, Patrik Henry Bass, Gregory Boyea, Trina Felder, Michele Griffin, Nazenet Habtezghi, Sheila Harris, Althea L. Honegan, Marsha Kelly, Jovanca Maitland, Edgerton Maloney, Starre Moss, Paul Nocera, Larry Ramo, Danielle Robinson, Mia Stokes, Noel Victorino, Wilhelmenia Weston, Darryl Wilson, Sharon Wynne

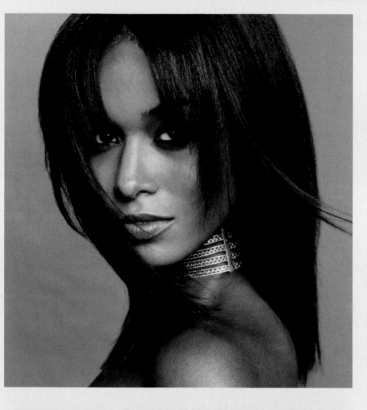

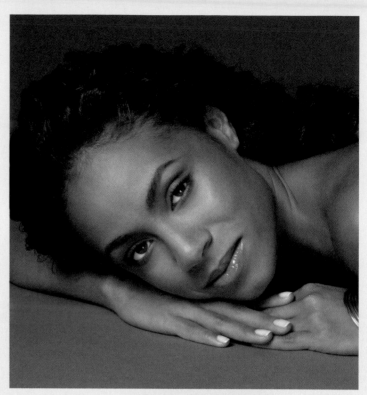

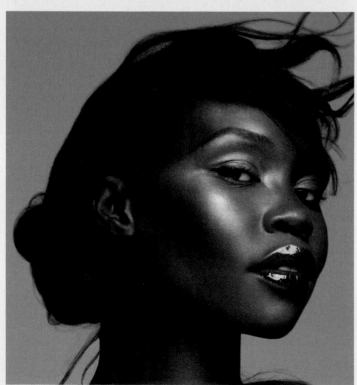

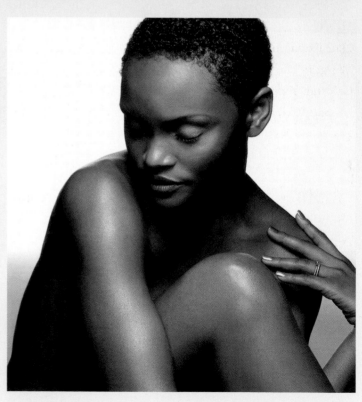

Contents

Beauty is...

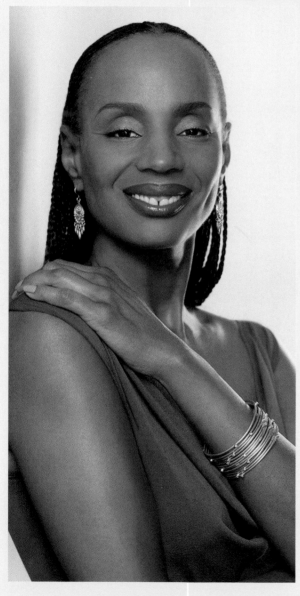

Ours. To exude and bask in. To imbibe, reflect and celebrate. It's more than skin-deep; it's soul and bone and unfathomed mystique, uncommon grace and confidence. Beauty is the light that shines through us as us.

Lean to lush, peach-complexioned to blueberry black, petite to towering, hair bone-straight to coiffed in our own natural way. Woman. Black woman. Goddess. Each of us a divine original. No less than the universe, we are the whole works.

But we have another image of ourselves, one that does not fit the facts. Tricked into believing there's a single ideal that appeals to every eye, we buy into, emulate and measure ourselves by a very narrow standard of beauty. "You're just not it," we've been taught. And so we object to ourselves; we embrace all these fallacies about what we are not, missing what should be most obvious: that there are six billion people on the planet, no two alike, each a marvel and miracle, each an expression of the Divine.

Each of us is a beauty. This was the starting point for *Beauty Basics & Beyond: 101 Ways to Keep Your Hair and Skin Fabulous*. The images, tips and techniques, the rituals and reflections—culled from the pages of ESSENCE and the experts we work with by editor Patricia Hinds—are offered here to help us make the most of the physical gifts that God has given us, to call attention to what we've got. Because we've already got it all.

All we really need is water and nourishment, exercise and rest, sun and a deep relationship with Spirit to help us create wellness, balance and serenity. But there's no reason we shouldn't enjoy changing our hair, wearing makeup—and not because we're trying to make up for anything missing. We're not trying to mask but to reveal. All the world's our stage; it's always changing. And so are we—changing how we choose to present ourselves. Changing for the pure fun of it.

Hey, Beauty! Feel at home with yourself. It's your stage and your world. This is the best time ever to be a Black woman. Make *your* statement.

—Susan L. Taylor

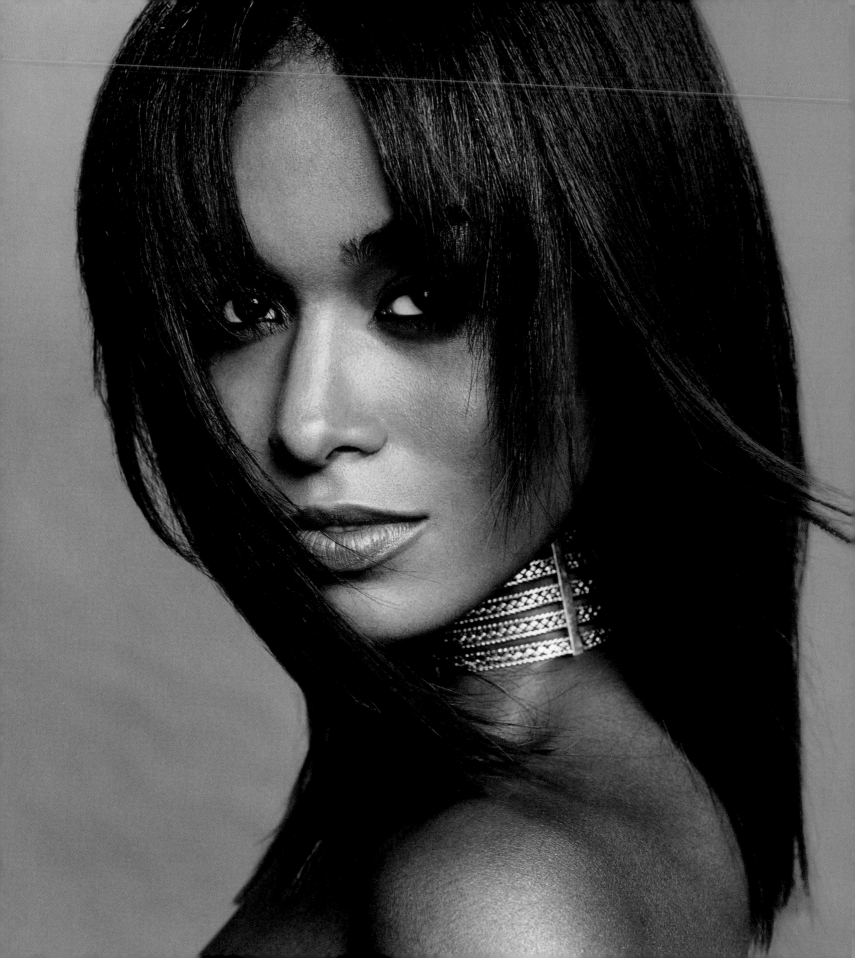

Loving Your Hair

Our hair, in all its diverse textures—from kinky to curly to wavy to straight—is truly one of the marvels of our race. Whether we celebrate the rhythm of our natural coils or opt for straighter styles, our options are greater than ever. Know your hair, the TLC your mane needs to stay healthy and luscious, and you can make every day a great-hair day.

Increase your use of moisturizing shampoos and conditioners to counteract the dehydration that is caused by the elements.

Whenever possible, apply a leave-in conditioner, especially on the ends, to keep frizzies and split ends in check.

Let go of that old-time adage about squeaky-clean hair. The truth is that squeaky hair means you've stripped hair of its natural oils.

Use hair color that mimics the colors of autumn with shades like copper, bronze and chestnut.

Hair Facts to Know

To keep your hair healthy and looking great, you have to know its strengths and weaknesses, what stresses it, and what it can and cannot do. Knowledge is power—and the more you know about the true nature and structure of your hair, the healthier it will become and the better you'll look and feel.

Structurally Speaking

Hair is composed of a chemical substance called keratin, a sulfur-rich protein that provides the hair with the strength it needs to withstand combing, brushing, heat and chemicals. The part of the hair that grows out of the scalp is the hair shaft or strand. Each strand of hair emerges from a tiny tubelike pit in the skin called a follicle, at the base of which is the papilla, the hair's source of blood, oxygen, other nutrients and new cells. As the cells in the papilla multiply to become an individual hair, they arrange themselves into three separate layers: the cuticle, the cortex and the medulla.

The cuticle, the outermost portion of the hair shaft, is composed of transparent, overlapping scalelike cells. Its main job is to protect the inner layers from moisture loss. Very curly or kinky hair has fewer cuticle layers than wavy and straight hair, and therefore, it is more fragile and vulnerable to heat and chemical damage. Each time you go for a touch-up or apply heat from a curling iron or blow-dryer, a degree of the moisture needed for softness and manageability is lost.

The cortex, which is just inside the cuticle, contains the pigment that gives your hair its color. This arrangement of cells is sensitive to chemicals and physical damage.

The medulla is the hair's innermost portion; it's a small core of cells that run the length of the hair shaft.

Assess Your Tresses

For your hair to look great and perform well, you must understand your two T's—texture and type—before beginning a hair-care regimen. Some of us have been relaxing our hair for so long that we've forgotten what our natural texture looks like.

Texture

Think of texture as your hair's true character, its natural shape and its original curl pattern—kinky, curly or wavy—without added chemicals and styling aids.

Quick Test: Just before getting a touch-up, pull out a few strands of hair close to your scalp from different places on your head. Place them on a white sheet of paper and notice how they look. If your hair is chemically relaxed, pull the strands and examine the new growth area only. The hairs might be loose and wavy, tightly curled or coiled like a spring. You may see that the

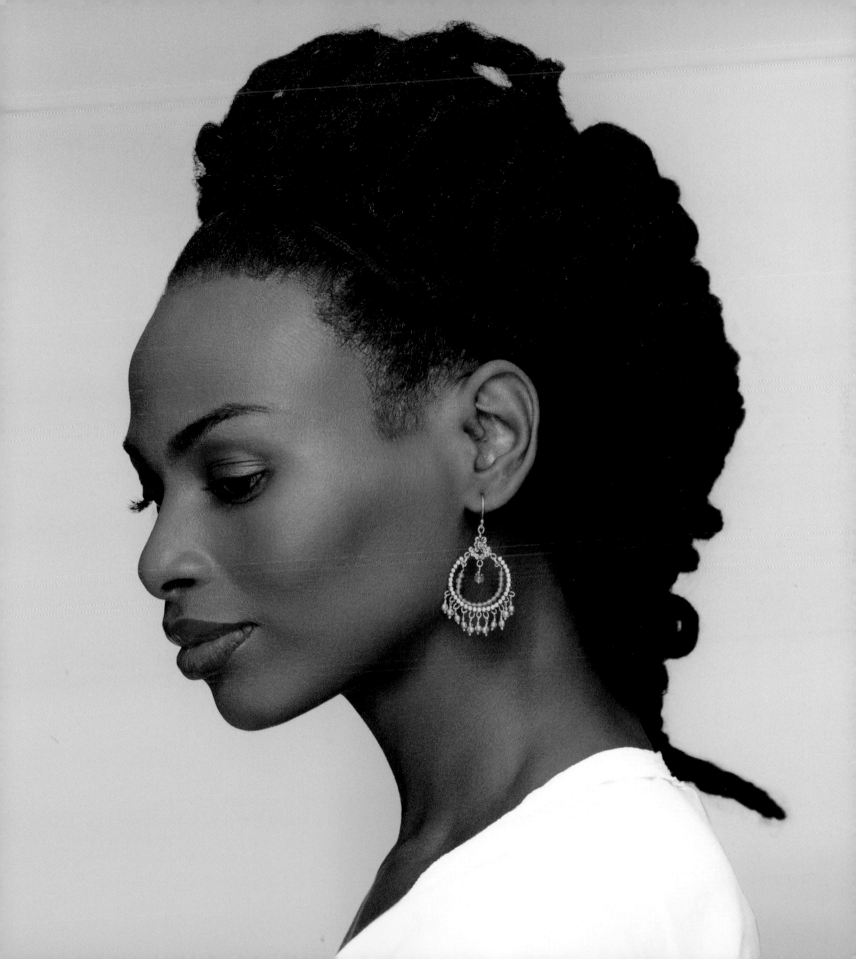

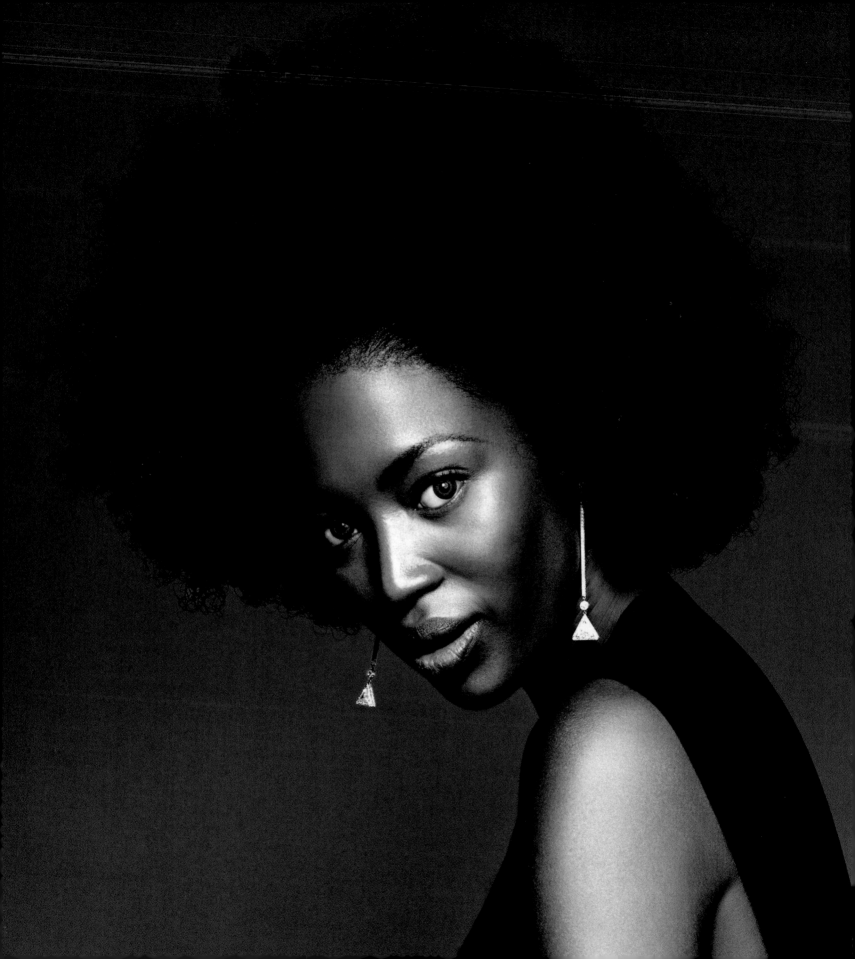

With relaxed or color-treated hair, frequent deep-oil and moisture conditioning is vital to maintain its health.

———

Feed your hair from the inside. Include these essential nutrients in your daily diet: omega-3 fatty acids (found in abundance in salmon and flaxseed oil); protein (found in soy and tofu, meat, poultry and dairy products); vitamins and minerals (found in fresh fruit and vegetables).

———

Cover hair with a silk scarf before bedtime to help your hair stay put and protect it from friction and breakage that can result from sleeping on a cotton pillowcase.

texture in the front differs slightly from the textures at the nape and crown. This is common. On average, we have at least two differing textures of hair on our head; hence, some sections of our hair are easier to manage, and some respond more quickly to chemicals, which can make them more prone to damage.

Type

Your hair type is determined by the diameter of the strands and typically belongs to one of three categories: fine, medium or coarse.

Quick Test: Examine the diameter of your individual strands. If the strands look wispy and thin, you have fine hair. If they are medium or thick in diameter, your hair is medium or coarse. Note: If your hair is healthy, you'll be able to slide your fingers down the shaft without any resistance.

Porosity

Black hair especially needs moisture to maintain its health. Porosity refers to the hair's ability to absorb moisture. As a rule, fine strands tend to be more porous, while coarse hair is usually not. The more porous your hair, the faster it absorbs chemicals—so you'll only need a short processing time for relaxers and color. This can be a good thing if you have a sensitive scalp, but it can also make the hair more vulnerable to damage from chemicals left on too long. On the flip side, it takes medium and coarse hair longer to "take" hair coloring and relaxers.

Quick Test: Separate a small section of hair at the front, and back-comb the strands as you do when teasing hair. Notice how the hair bunches up. If the hair bunches immediately, it is very porous or damaged; if the hair bunches up a little or not at all, it is healthy or less porous.

Elasticity

Elasticity refers to the hair's ability to stretch and return to its original length without breaking. Healthy hair should be able to stretch about one-fifth of its length when dry and one-half of its length when wet.

Quick Test: Select a hair strand and hold it between the index fingers and thumbs of both hands. Gently pull the strand. If it stretches easily and returns to its original length, you've got good elasticity. If the strand breaks or doesn't return, then your hair needs lots more TLC. Poor elasticity is an indication of chemical damage and that you may be overusing heated appliances, relaxers or coloring.

Growing, Growing, Gone

Basically, there are three stages in the life cycle of each hair on our body. A hair is born, matures, then dies. Hair is in the first stage, called anagen, about four to six years. About 80 to 90 percent of the hair on your scalp is in this stage. In the second stage, the catagen phase, hair ceases to grow, or "rests," for about two to three weeks. Before transitioning into the final stage, the telogen phase, where it sheds naturally (notice we didn't say break), we lose 50 to 100 hairs per day.

Your Hair Hook-Up Guide

With a better understanding of your hair texture and type, you can customize a nourishing hair-care regimen that's tailor-made for you. All hair types need moisture and oil. The amounts will vary according to your type and texture, which is the natural pattern of your hair, free from chemicals.

If Your Natural Hair Is Kinky & Fine

Your hair is probably dry and fragile and gets a bit of frizz even if it's relaxed. Your hair is so precious and fragile, you'll need moisture, oil and protein to prevent damage and breakage. Stressless low-maintenance styles are best for your tresses. If you choose to relax your strands, opt for a mild formula. Your relaxed hair will need more moisture—from conditioners, hot-oil treatments and daily moisturizers—than if you leave it natural.

- **Best Shampoo:** Choose volumizing moisturizing shampoos that contain thickeners to give hair a fuller appearance.
- **Best Conditioner:** Opt for a protein-rich moisturizing formula and a nourishing leave-in conditioner to strengthen the hair. Use a deep-conditioning or hot-oil treatment twice a month.

If Your Natural Hair Is Kinky & Medium

The versatility of your hair allows you to have completely different styles from day to day. It's not as fragile as fine hair, but it also has a tendency to get frizzy. It can be relaxed gently to leave body in the hair but also to give it the flexibility of wearing natural, curly or straight looks.

- **Best Shampoo:** Regular maintenance includes a moisturizing shampoo once a week.
- **Best Conditioner:** Use a leave-in conditioner before styling and an intensive conditioning treatment twice a month.

If Your Natural Hair Is Kinky & Coarse

Because of its density, kinky and coarse hair can require more oil and moisturizers. Because it is stronger than other hair types, when it comes to styling, you can do it all—you can wear it natural, press and curl it, or relax it.

- **Best Shampoo:** Use a moisture-rich shampoo or a shampoo for dry hair.
- **Best Conditioner:** Each week, apply a protein-based and moisturizing conditioner to maintain elasticity, and a nourishing leave-in formula to add strength; and use a hot-oil treatment once or twice a month.

If Your Natural Hair Is Curly & Fine

This type is soft and fragile. It looks great natural and requires only a minimum amount of heat to make it straight, if that's your choice. Since this hair is often dry, too much heat will quickly cause damage, and applying a relaxer will reduce body. There are two ways to loosen your curls: temporarily by pressing it straight or permanently by applying the mildest relaxer for just a few minutes. Experts say that constant use of excessive heat can weaken and permanently straighten the hairs or loosen the natural curls, making them limp and wavy instead of curly.

- **Best Shampoo:** Use a moisturizing shampoo.
- **Best Conditioner:** Choose a leave-in conditioner (watery in consistency) to moisturize hair without weighing it down, and use a deep conditioner at least every two weeks for added moisture and strength.

If Your Natural Hair Is Curly & Medium

This hair type does not need a relaxer to become straight. You can blow-dry and use a flat iron or press with a hot comb for a sleek look.

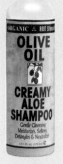

• *Best Shampoo:* Use a detangling shampoo containing ingredients like soy protein, which smoothes the hair's surface, making it easier to comb out snarls and knots.
• *Best Conditioner:* A silicone-based conditioner can be used for sheen, coating the cuticles and reducing frizz. A protein-based conditioner will strengthen strands.

If Your Natural Hair Is Curly & Coarse

This hair has a strong curl pattern and a tendency to become dry if it isn't regularly moisturized. With an oil-based moisturizing gel applied to wet hair, your natural curl will be enhanced for an easy, curly look. For a straight, sleek finish, blow-dry while using a large round brush, or use a flat iron or a hot comb after blow-drying. A mild relaxer works well if you want to keep your hair straight permanently.

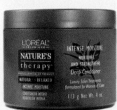

• *Best Shampoo:* Stick to a moisturizing shampoo with humectants that pull moisture from the air.

• *Best Conditioner:* Use a leave-in conditioner after each shampoo and a deep moisturizing conditioner every two weeks; apply a hot-oil treatment once a month.

If Your Natural Hair Is Wavy & Fine

Your hair, which can be oily, is great worn natural. Just a bit of heat turns it from wavy to sleek. You have multiple styling options—from naturally wavy to soft curly to straight looks.

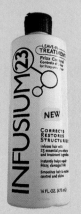

• *Best Shampoo:* Wash every three to four days with a clarifying shampoo.
• *Best Conditioner:* Use a lightweight leave-in conditioner to enhance your natural waves.

If Your Natural Hair Is Wavy & Medium

Natural hair is perfect for you. Blowouts and a flat iron or hot-comb press will achieve a straight look. Humid weather often causes hair to frizz, so relaxing is a great option if you want your hair to stay straight.

• *Best Shampoo:* Invest in a mild, antifrizz shampoo.
• *Best Conditioner:* Your hair will look great with deep conditioning twice a month and a hot-oil treatment once a month.

If Your Natural Hair Is Wavy & Coarse

Wear it natural or straighten it easily using a blow-dryer with a round brush, flat iron or a hot comb. To permanently straighten your curl, you can apply a mild relaxer. You can get great naturally wavy styles. Just massage a light gel into your freshly shampooed and conditioned hair. Then attach a diffuser to your blow-dryer, and use low heat to dry your hair.

• *Best Shampoo:* Your hair has a tendency to tangle, so use a detangling and moisturizing shampoo.
• *Best Conditioner:* Use moisturizing and protein-based conditioners to maintain strength and elasticity.

If your scalp is dry and flaky, use a dandruff-control shampoo, and let it sit for about five minutes before massaging and rinsing.

For dry hair, use a hot-oil treatment at least once a month.

Basic Hair Care

Healthy, great-looking hair is the goal, and it's an achievable one. Remember your strands are inherently delicate, so don't stress them. Harsh chemicals, excessive heat, sun, chlorine and sweat can cause dryness and damage. Shampooing, conditioning and styling are the building blocks of manageable, beautiful hair. Armed with the following information, you'll be in control of your crown, whether you regularly go to a pro or do it yourself at home.

Shampooing

Not all shampoos are created equal. Make sure you choose one designed for your hair's specific needs—hydrating, clarifying, smoothing or volumizing. Keep your scalp healthy, and wash your hair at least every week to ten days. This is so important for sisters wearing braids and weaves, which can easily trap oils, product buildup, pollution and bacteria. Lather up two or three times and massage your scalp using the balls of your fingertips, and don't scratch your scalp. Rinse thoroughly. An itchy scalp may signal dryness, a need to shampoo more frequently or a condition that needs a dermatologist's attention. Experts caution against shampooing hair until it's squeaky clean, which will rob your hair of natural oils.

Types of Shampoos

➤ **Hydrating**—to add moisture
➤ **Clarifying**—to remove excess oil and product buildup
➤ **Smoothing**—to control frizz
➤ **Volumizing**—to add body and fullness

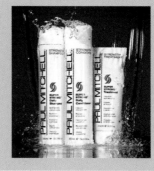

Types of Conditioners

➤ **Protein-based**—maintains strength and elasticity
➤ **Hot-oil treatment**—lubricates hair
➤ **Moisturizing**—adds moisture for flexibility and hydration

Conditioning

After shampooing, always follow up with a conditioner to replenish moisture and strengthen hair. Use a treatment best suited for your hair's texture, type and present condition. There are several types of conditioners:

Deep conditioners are formulated to penetrate the hair shaft. They strengthen, moisturize and lubricate. They are effective on the inner and outer structure of the hair. This type of conditioner usually takes 15 to 20 minutes under heat to penetrate the hair.

Instant conditioners are rinsed out after a few minutes. They are used for detangling and softening hair and to close the cuticle, making hair easier to comb.

Leave-in conditioners give added moisture and nourishment, and they act as a protectant before drying and heat-styling.

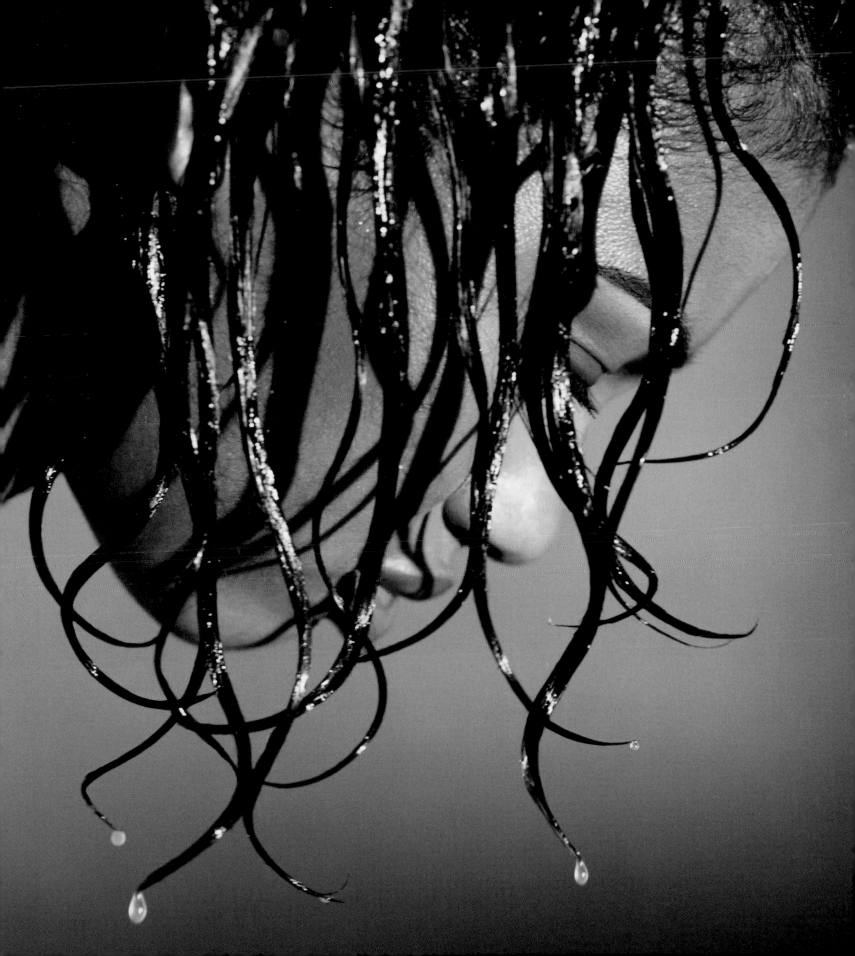

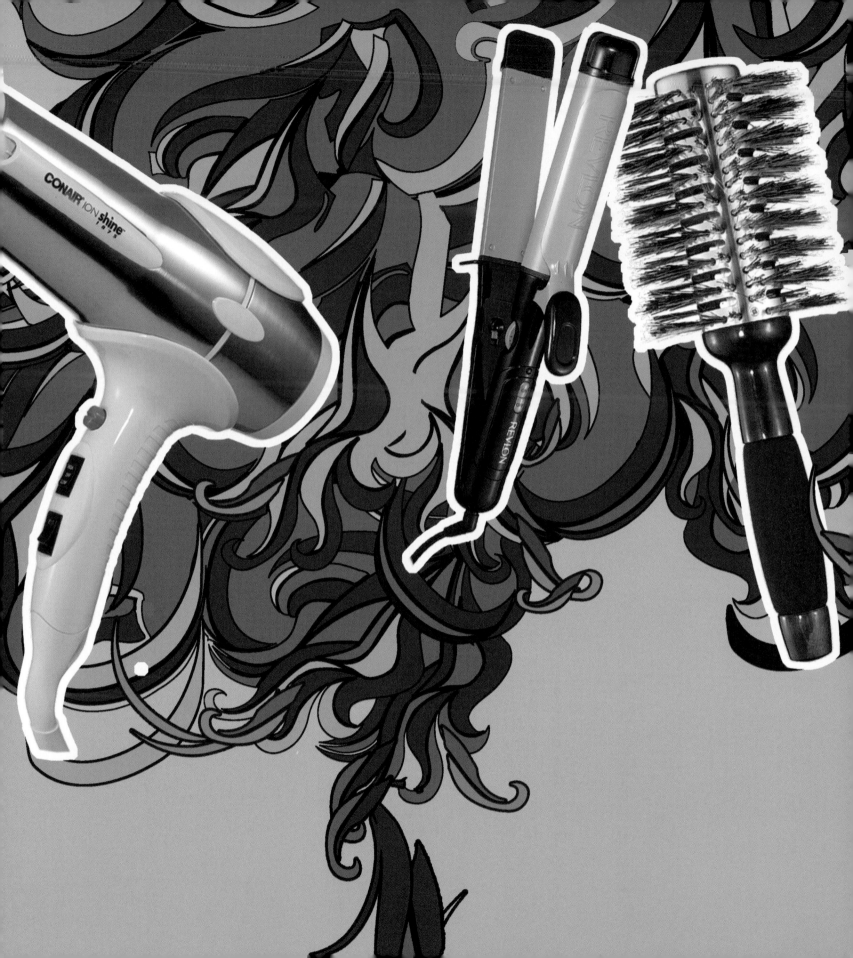

Natural oils, such as olive, sesame and palma christi oil, when combined with most hair products, penetrate and protect the hair shaft. Add a few drops of oil to your relaxer and colorants.

Since drying with heat and styling with curling irons are probably part of your hair-care routine, protect your hair with a moisturizing cream before applying any heat.

Styling: Drying Your Hair

There are a few ways to dry your hair—with a hand-held blow-dryer (with or without diffuser), a hooded dryer, a towel or by air-drying. Since air-drying is heat- and stress-free, it's the healthiest hair-drying technique. On a whole, heat-styling is hard enough on hair, but using the wrong technique makes it worse. That's why starting with healthy hair is so important!

10 Tips for Blow-Drying

Always keep in mind the four T's when blow-drying your hair: treatment (rub on a moisturizing lotion to protect your hair), temperature control (keep it low to medium heat), tension (don't stretch or stress wet hair) and technique (keep the blower moving and about 2 to 3 inches from your hair)—and you won't damage your locks. Here's how to safely blow-dry your mane:

1 Detangle your hair with a large-toothed comb, starting from the ends to the scalp before blow-drying. Combing from the scalp can cause breakage.

2 Treat hair with a lightweight barrier such as a leave-in conditioner, antifrizz serum or heat-activated styling lotion before blow-drying, to protect it against heat and help smooth the cuticle, which will boost shine.

3 Dry your hair in sections, starting at the nape, moving toward the top.

4 Avoid overheating the hair by sitting under a dryer for 10 to 15 minutes to remove excess water before using a blow-dryer. It's easier to get a smoother, shinier finish if you blow-dry hair that's already about 80 percent dry.

5 To avoid scorching your hair, keep the dryer moving, and avoid placing the dryer directly on your hair (1,500 watts is sufficient for home use).

6 Use a comb attachment or a round brush if your hair is healthy, strong and coarse. Avoid using comb attachments and round brushes on chemically treated hair.

7 Blow the hair in a downward motion. This causes the cuticle to lay flat and reflect light, giving strands a supershiny appearance.

8 Avoid excessive heat along your hairline, which is usually fine and vulnerable to damage.

9 Give your hair a blast of cool air after applying intense heat. Hot air opens the cuticles, and cool air closes them, which seals in moisture.

10 Add a diffuser to your dryer if you want to keep your kinky, curly or wavy hair texture.

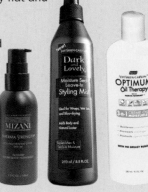

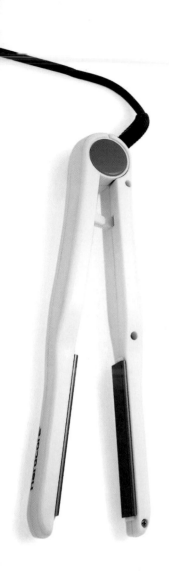

Curl Power

With the help of rollers, hot rollers, curling irons, pins and even rods, you can achieve anything from a slight bend to a riot of saucy curls. Before using hot rollers or a curling iron, apply a protective moisture cream to shield strands from heat and boost shine. Most textures don't need to go higher than the medium setting on your thermostat-controlled curling iron.

Curling Irons

➤ **Barrel Iron** (small, medium and large)
   Best Use: Create small ringlets to big, bouncy curls or waves.
➤ **Crimper** (small, medium and large)
   Best Use: Get a crimplike pattern (think ripples of waves) on hair.
➤ **Flat Iron** (mini, medium and large)
   Best Use: Straighten bangs and curl, smooth or style all lengths of hair.
➤ **C Iron**
   Best use: Give hair a little bend with a C iron.

Roller Sets

Roller sets are easiest on your hair and the way to set long-lasting curls. But all rollers are not created equal. The size of your roller will determine the tightness and size of your curl. The most popular are rods, magnetic and wire mesh.

Rollers (rod, magnetic and wire mesh)
How to Use: Section freshly shampooed and conditioned hair, and wrap ends smoothly with end paper. Roll the hair toward the scalp, and depending on the type of roller, pin to hold, then dry under a hooded dryer.
Dry Time: You'll need 30 to 60 minutes for drying; wire mesh rollers only need up to 45 minutes for hair to dry.

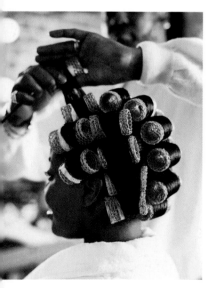

How to Do the Perfect Wrap

1. Shampoo and condition your hair.
2. Work lotion through your hair.
3. Comb and smooth your hair around scalp clockwise or counterclockwise, depending on how you plan for your style to fall and the effect you want.
4. Place a wrapping tissue around your hairline to secure hair in place.
5. Sit under the dryer for about 30 to 45 minutes (or until it's dry).
6. Remove wrap and comb your hair out. Apply a protective moisture cream or silicone-based lotion.
7. You can leave your hair in this straight look or style your hair with a flat or curling iron, depending on the desired effect.
Note: For wrapping dry hair, use bobby pins or clips and a silk scarf to secure hair before bedtime.

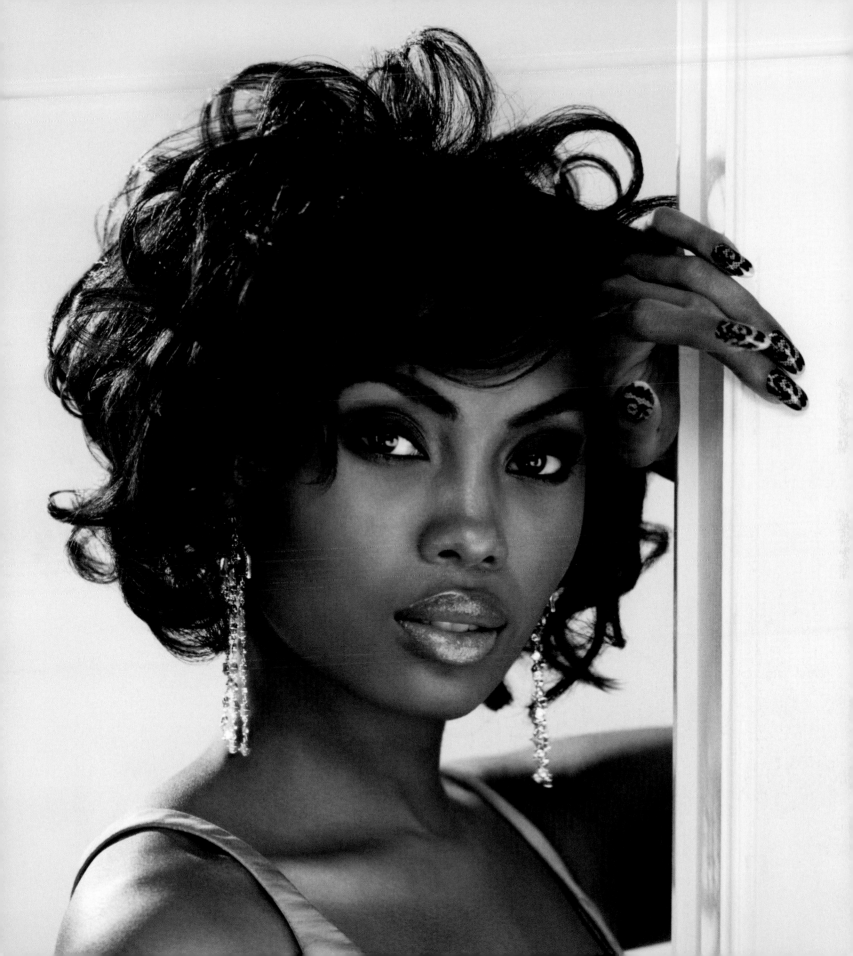

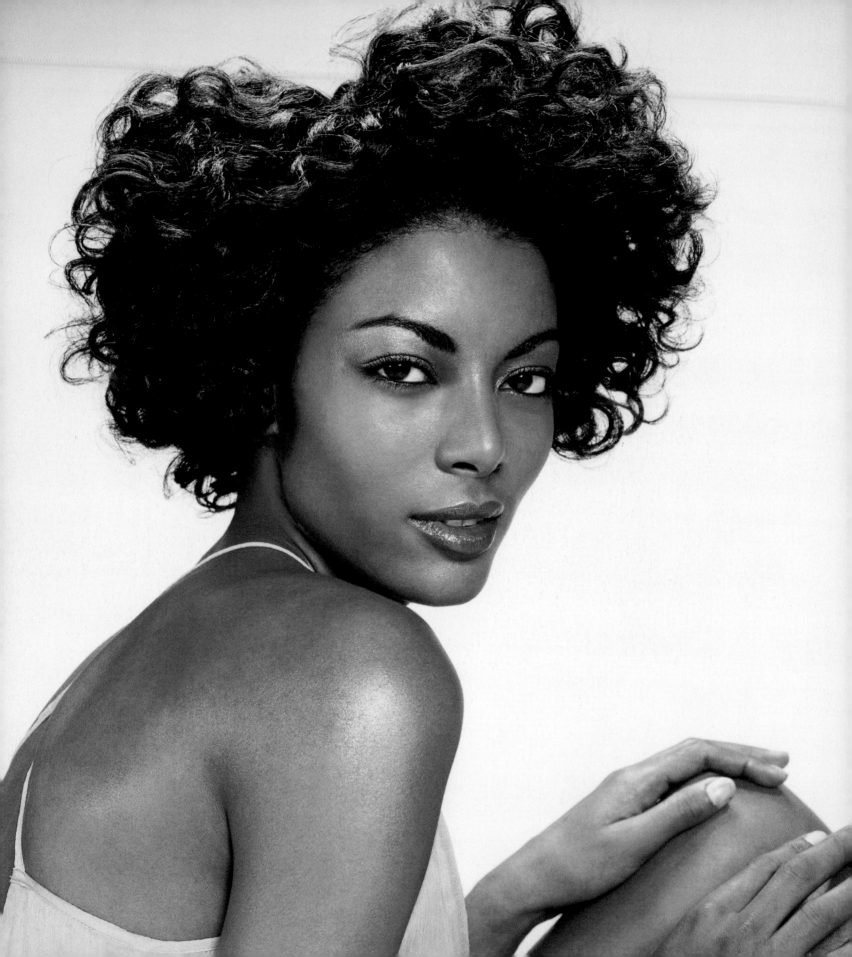

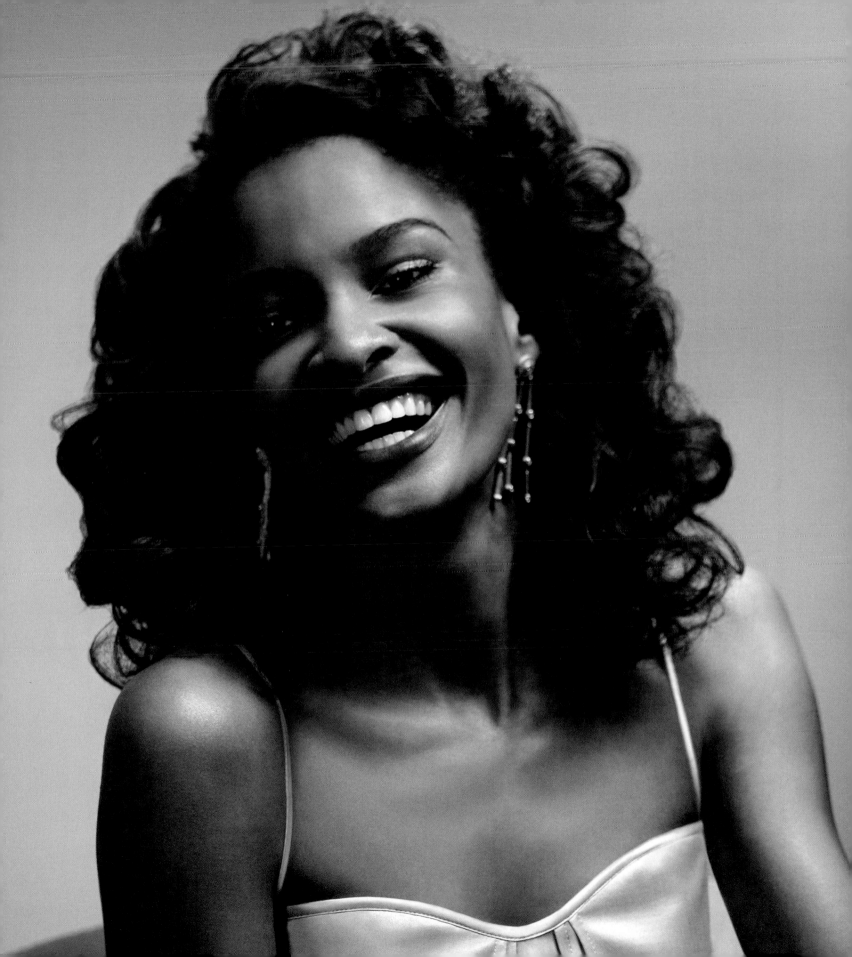

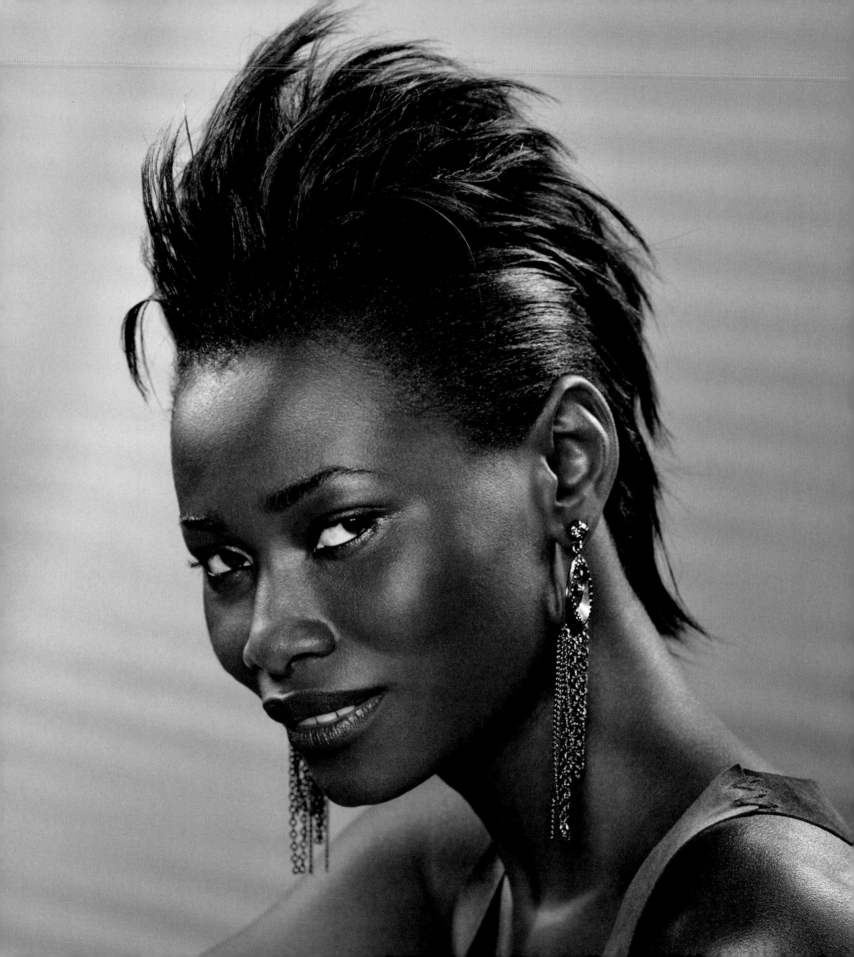

Styling Aids

Every sister can have hypnotically attractive hair. Styling aids can be used with blow-drying, roller setting and wrapping. Here are the specialized products for your hair texture, type and style.

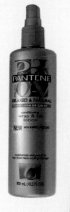

Setting Lotion

What It Is: Setting lotion is a liquid styling aid.

Purpose: It gives hair long-term styling memory. It's especially effective in helping hair roller set keep its curl.

Wrapping Lotion

What It Is: This aid is a lightweight, nonalcohol liquid styling formula.

Purpose: It softens hair and provides light hold.

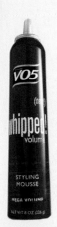

Mousse

What It Is: This is a light-hold, fast-drying foam.

Purpose: Mousse creates volume and is a boon for fine hair.

Hair Spray

What It Is: A pump or aerosol liquid formula, hair spray provides hold.

Purpose: It keeps hair in place and adds some shine.

Gel

What It Is: Used on wet hair, gel is a thick styling formula.

Purpose: It provides firm hold for definition of curls and smoothes edges between touch-ups.

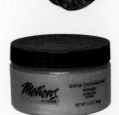

Glaze

What It Is: Glaze is a thick styling aid used on dry hair.

Purpose: It holds hair in place and adds shine. Use glaze for sculpting wet looks, smoothing your hairline and maintaining curly or spiky looks.

Wax or Pomade

What It Is: Wax or pomade, a heavy, sometimes sticky styling aid, provides the most holding power.

Purpose: It separates and holds curly and spiky styles.

Moisturizers

Hydrating your hair is an essential part of your maintenance ritual. Here are three types to take a shine to:

Oil

What It Is: Oil for hair is a substance composed of natural or synthetic lightweight moisturizers.

Purpose: It softens the hair's outer layer and allows moisture to penetrate deeply. Natural oils such as jojoba and palma christi complement your hair's natural oils. Silicone-based formulas can clog your scalp's pores. Both types can be used for natural and relaxed tresses. Since your scalp produces its own oils, adding more can attract dirt, clog the scalp's pores and stunt hair growth. One of the biggest mistakes many sisters make is overusing oil-based products, which will just look greasy.

Spray Sheen

What It Is: This is an oil that usually comes in a spray or pump container.

Purpose: As its name indicates, it adds shine to hair.

Moisturizing or Dressing Cream

What It Is: This is a light cream or lotion.

Purpose: This aid infuses hair with moisturizers and protects it from the elements. It also imparts shine and protects hair from damage when using heated tools and appliances.

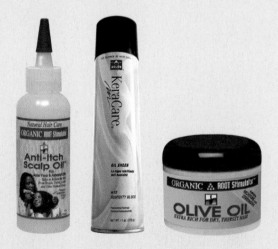

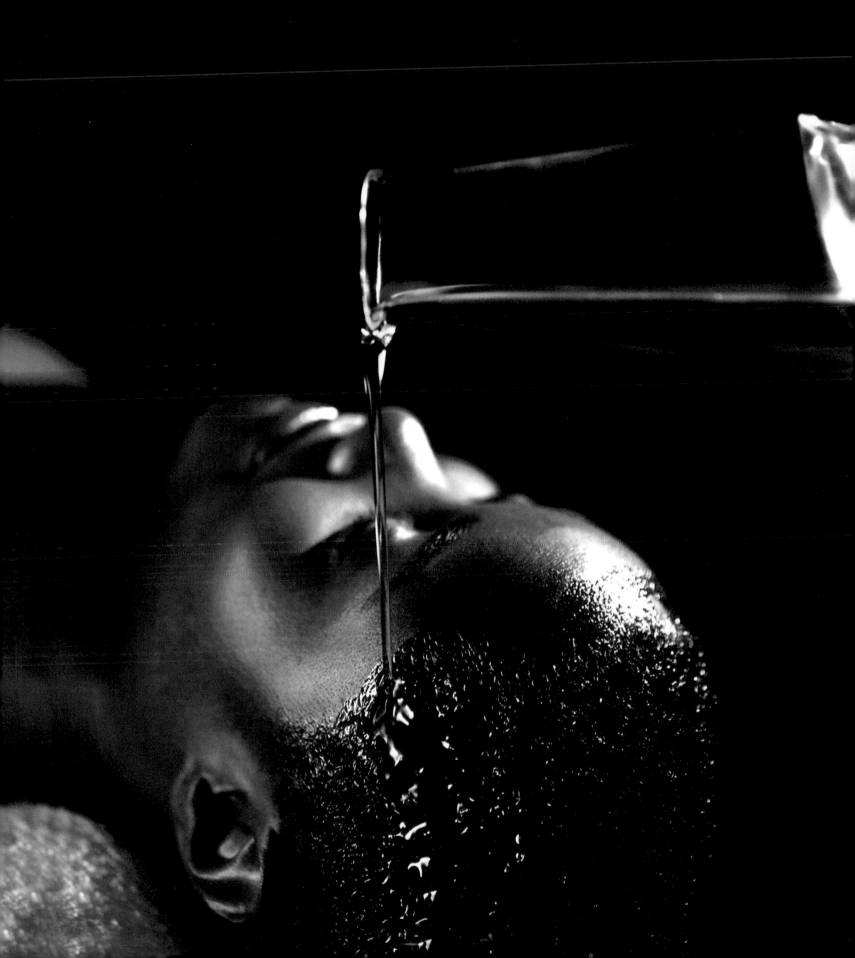

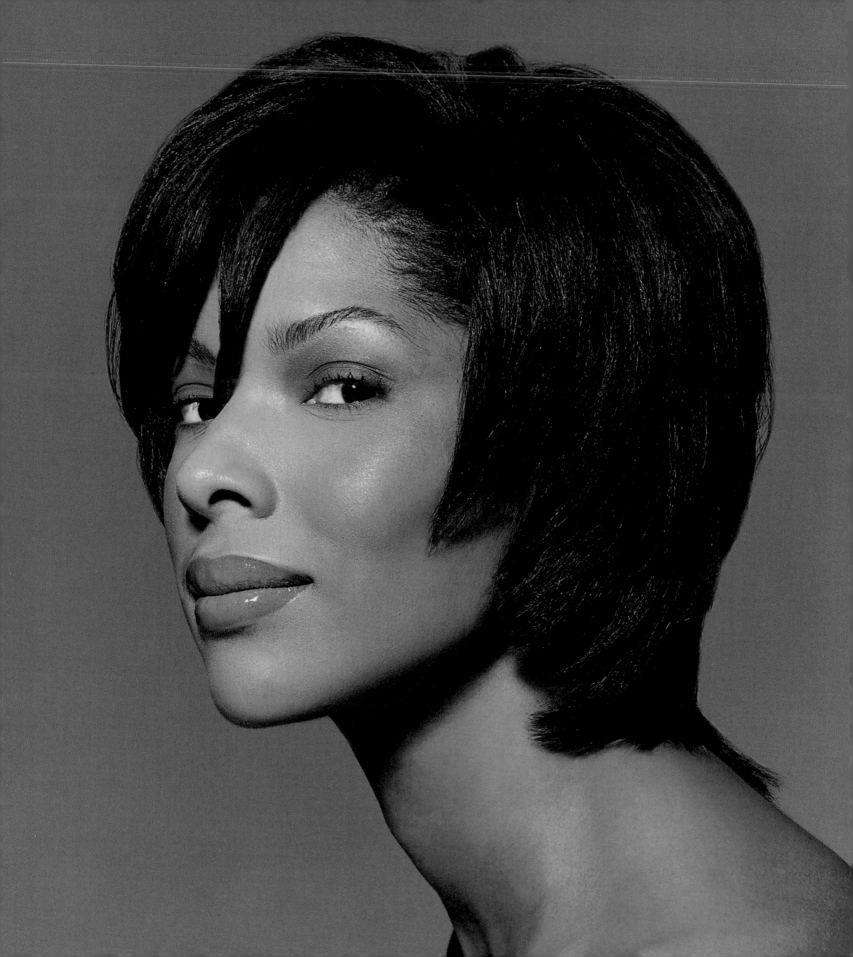

Getting Straight: Relaxed-Hair Care

Although technological advances over the past decade have greatly improved relaxer formulas and made them less harsh, relaxing the hair without damaging it requires great skill. Unless you're expert at it or have a sisterfriend who is, you should put your hair in the hands of a professional. But whether the treatment is done at home or in a salon, make sure that only a formulation created for your hair texture and type touches your mane. Here's what's on the market.

Lye Relaxer

➤ **How It Works:** The active ingredient—sodium hydroxide (lye)—breaks down the hydrogen and sulfide bonds that give the hair its shape. Smoothing the product through your hair rearranges the bonds, straightening the hair.

➤ **Best Used On:** Choose this formulation if your hair is not subjected to any other chemical processes.

➤ **Pros:** It straightens the hair, which offers styling versatility.

➤ **Cons:** A lye relaxer can cause irritation and burns if left on the scalp too long. Overprocessing causes hair damage, breakage and possibly permanent bald spots.

Straightening Balm

➤ **How It Works:** A straightening balm is made out of a combination of silicones, plant extracts, amino acids or wheat protein; it is applied to wet hair prior to blowing it dry. Then heat from a ceramic flat iron smoothes hair cuticles and seals in shine.

➤ **Best Used On:** Moderately curly and wavy hair best benefit from this styling aid.

➤ **Pros:** Straightening balm offers a quick and simple way to achieve a straight look—sans chemicals.

➤ **Cons:** It is not long-lasting—moisture causes hair to revert.

No-Lye Relaxer

➤ **How It Works:** Although the active ingredient—calcium hydroxide—is called no-lye, it is still lye. It breaks down the hydrogen and sulfide bonds that give the hair its shape and rearranges the hair bonds.

➤ **Best Used On:** A no-lye relaxer is an option for sisters whose scalp is sensitive or who use a permanent coloring agent, although it is not recommended by many experts. This formulation is best on hair that just needs its curl loosened a bit.

➤ **Pros:** It allows you to color and relax your hair, but never do both at the same time. Space these processes at least two weeks apart. Only a top-notch professional can handle the dual processes well, and only women with well-conditioned and coarse hair should opt for both.

➤ **Cons:** This type of relaxer deposits additional calcium on the hair, making it more prone to dryness and breakage. Plus, it won't completely straighten supertight hair, which leaves the shaft more porous and susceptible to damage. For this reason, many experts do not use this product.

Texturizer

➤ **How It Works:** It is created with activating lye used in lye-based relaxers. In fact, you can achieve a "texturized" look by simply leaving a lye-based relaxer on the hair for a shorter time.

➤ **Best Used On:** A texturizer is good for natural curls, which get loosened without totally breaking down their configuration.

➤ **Pro:** It tends to be less damaging to hair.

➤ **Con:** Achieving a straighter style requires using tools at higher temperatures.

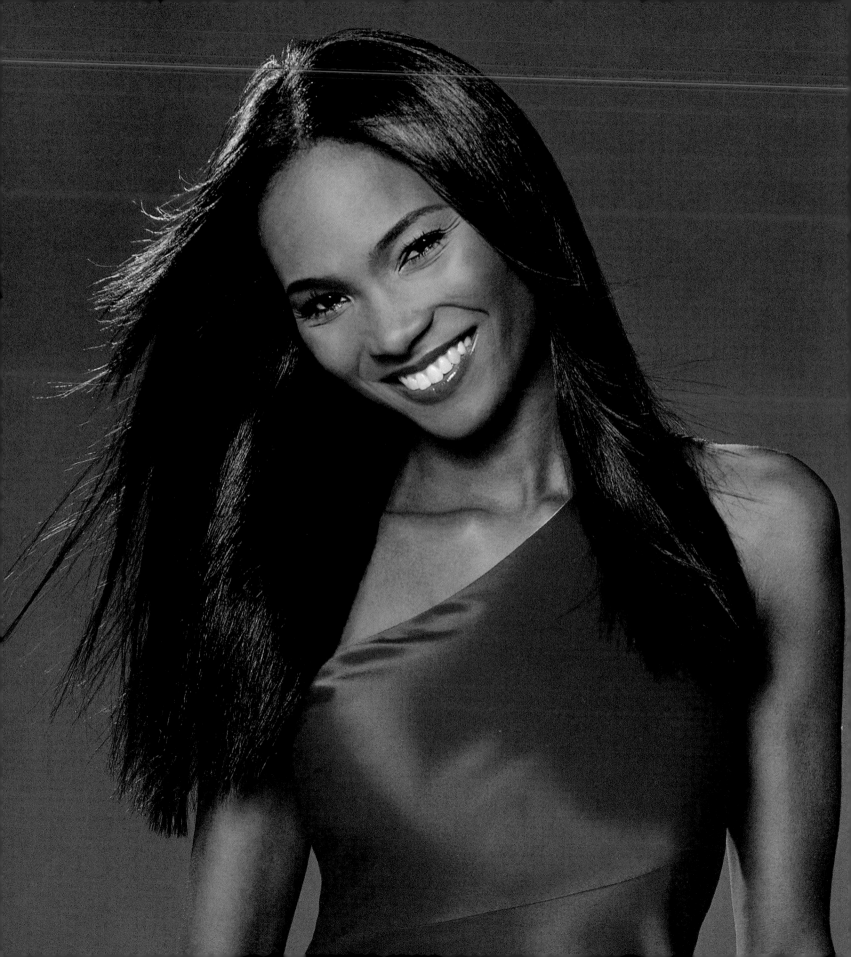

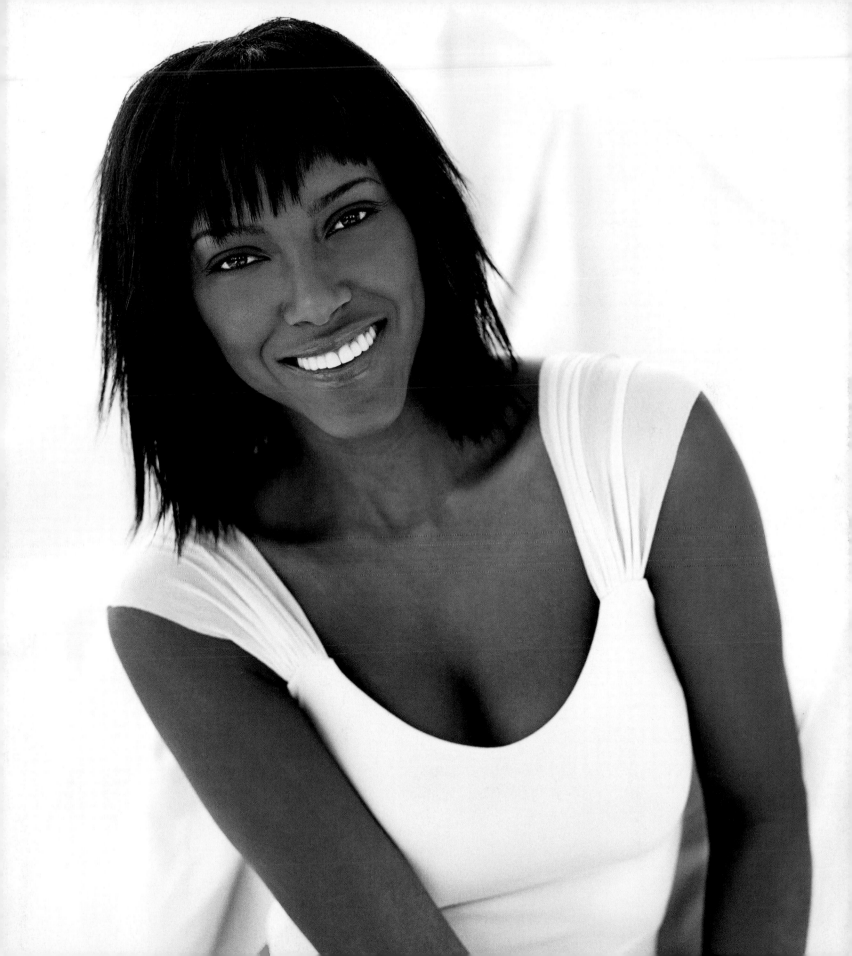

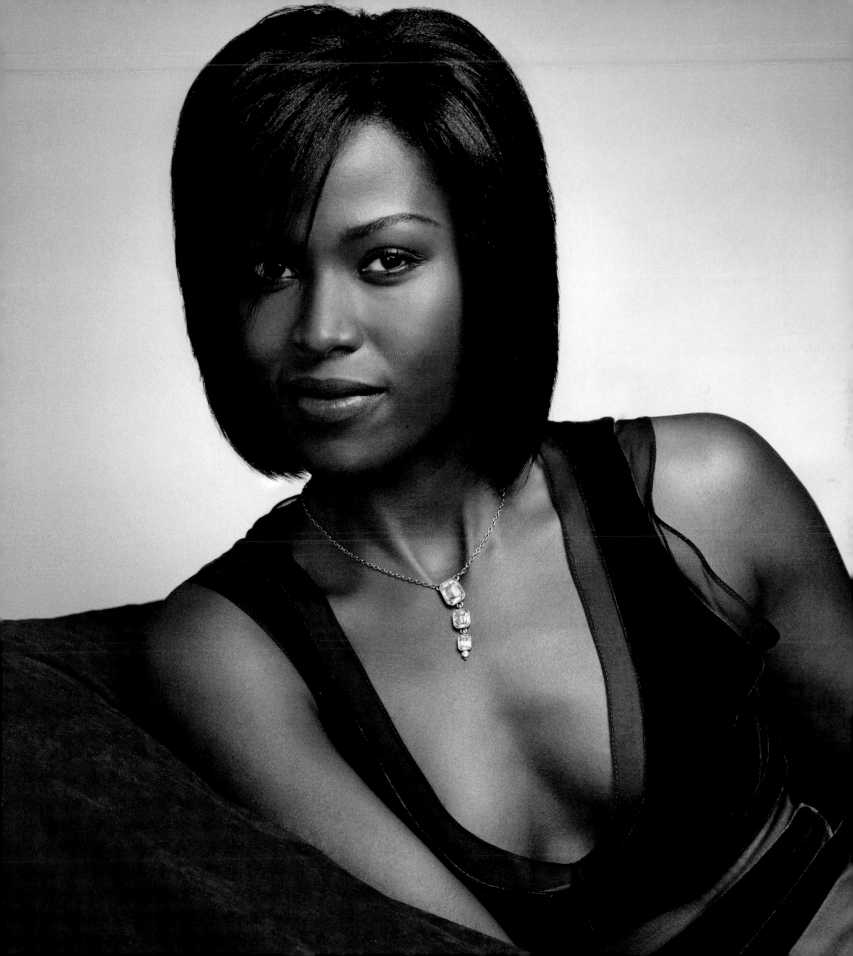

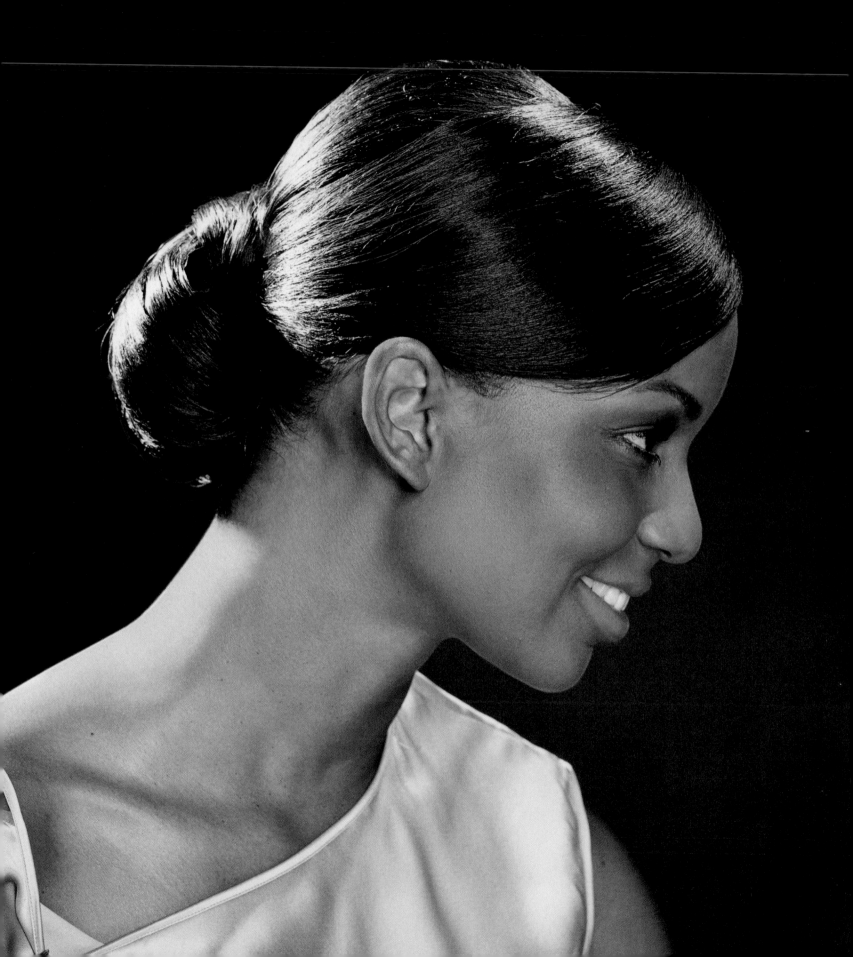

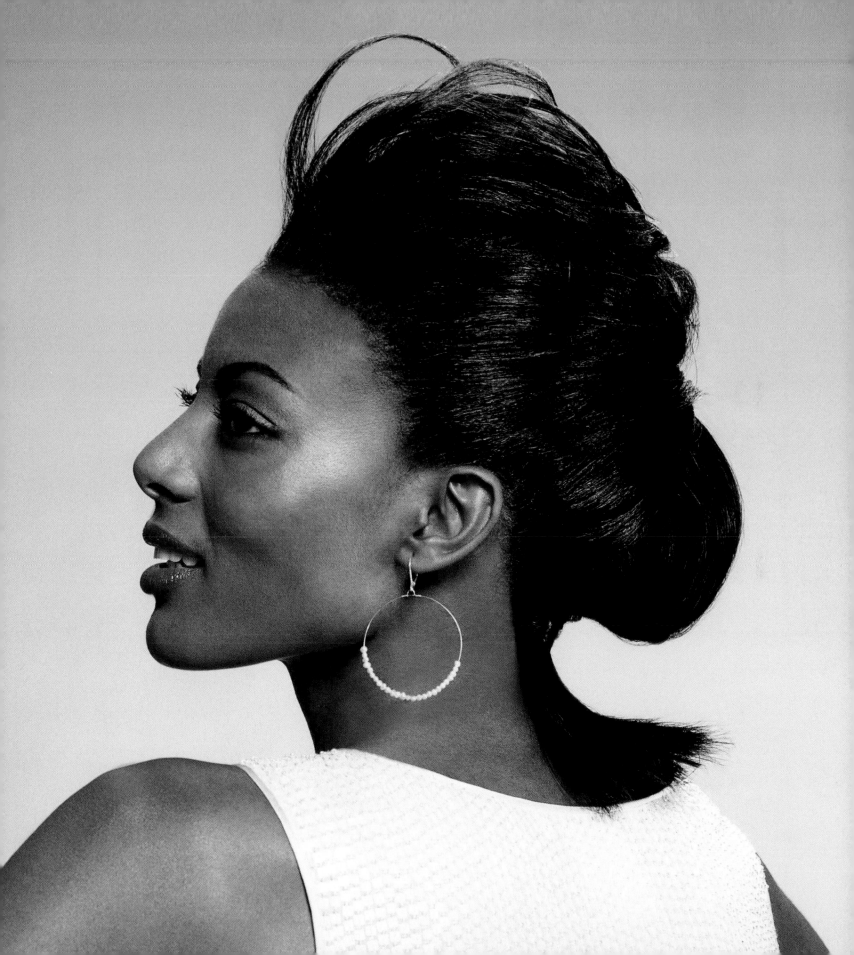

Relaxed-Hair Time Line

DAY TO DAY

Stimulate the scalp. Use the tips of your fingers (not your nails) to massage the scalp. Don't ever scratch your scalp or brush it 48 hours before a touch-up.

Keep it light. Use a spray sheen or light dressing cream to refresh your hair's shine.

Pay attention. Each day while styling your hair, notice how it performs—whether it's shedding excessively, feels dry or oily and what treatments and tools help it look spectacular. Get to know your hair intimately.

Avoid tension and friction. Use a covered band, not a tight rubber band, for your ponytail, and change its position regularly. Don't pull your hair taut. If you wear a part, switch it up now and then. And tie your hair up with a silk scarf at night to avoid damage—caused by friction from tossing and turning while you sleep.

WEEK TO WEEK

Alternate conditioning treatments. To ensure that your hair gets the proper balance of protein and moisture, alternate weekly treatments between protein and moisturizing conditioners or hot-oil and deep conditioners.

MONTH TO MONTH

Stay trimmed. Split ends ruin any style and compromise the health of your hair. So when you go in for your touch-ups every four to eight weeks, also have your ends trimmed.

Invest in quality products. Between salon visits, use the products, tools and techniques your stylist recommends. This will help ensure a salon finish at home.

Do It Yourself: Relaxers

Most of us have morphed into a kitchen beautician at one time or another, cutting, coloring or relaxing our hair at home. While salon professionals frown upon applying chemicals at home, manufacturers have provided the tools to do it yourself. If you choose to apply a relaxer at home, experts agree that you should take some precautions to avoid overprocessing and damaging your hair or scalp.

Begin with the right formula—mild, regular or super, based on what's best for your hair type and texture. If you overprocess your hair, it will become dry and brittle, and the strands will snap easily. See the beginning of this chapter to determine your hair type and texture.

Have a friend on hand to help. Relaxing requires quick and thorough application. Since you can't see every angle of your head, it's best to have someone to assist you in applying the relaxer uniformly.

Protect the scalp, hairline, ears and nape. Apply a shea-butter base to protect the skin and alleviate the burning and irritation relaxers sometimes cause. Be sure to distribute the protective base evenly on the scalp. Using too much can actually compromise the relaxer's effectiveness. Lightly dab on a small amount with your fingers, or use a pointed-nozzle squirt bottle for precise application. Avoid putting base on your hair, because it slows the activation of the relaxer.

Wear plastic gloves. Protect your hands. The chemicals in relaxers can irritate your skin.

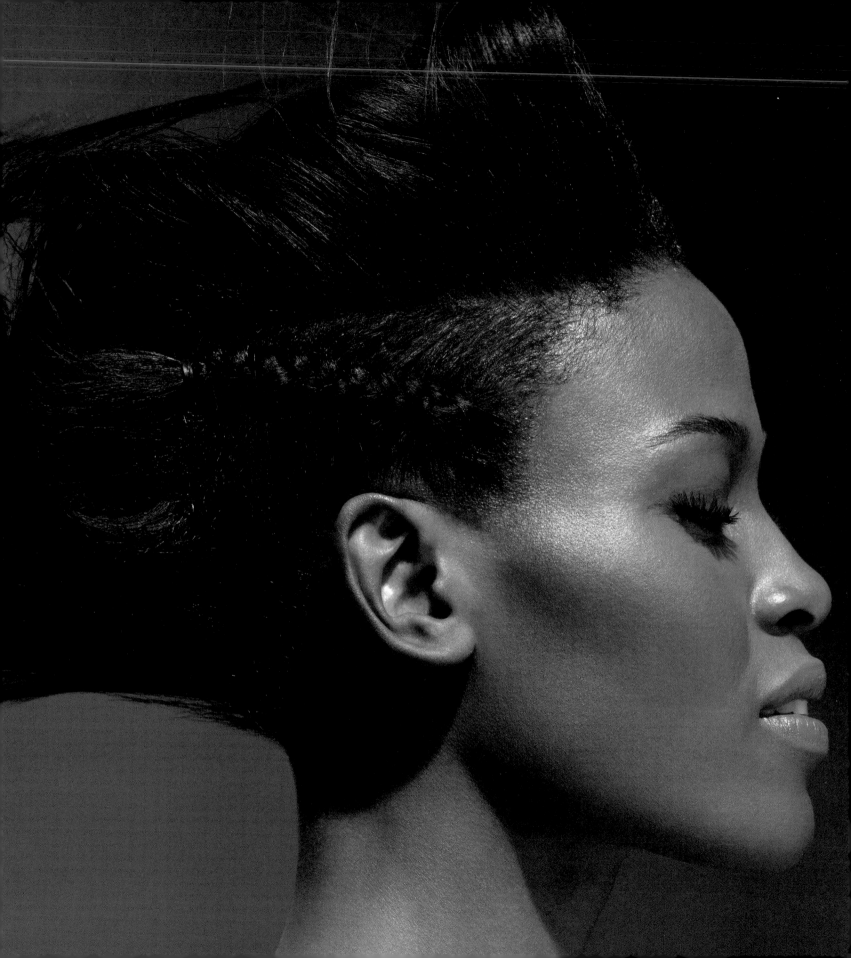

Don't touch up too soon. Make sure you have at least a half an inch of new growth. Otherwise, you're exposing your hair to chemicals it doesn't need yet.

Make sure your scalp is healthy. Don't relax your hair if you a have a sore, scab or scratch on your scalp. Relaxers are for topical use only, and you don't want the chemicals to enter your body.

Avoid scratching your scalp prior to relaxing. The chemicals can irritate the scalp and enter your system.

Don't shampoo or wet your hair 24 hours prior to application. Your natural oils and the top layer of your scalp help protect it from the chemicals.

Prevent overprocessing. Apply a moisturizing conditioner to previously relaxed hair as a protective barrier. Avoid overlapping and relax only new growth.

Start at the nape. The hair in the back of your head tends to be most resistant.

Apply to your hairline last. It's usually the finest, thinnest and most prone to breakage.

Apply the relaxer carefully. Use your gloved fingertips, an application brush or squeeze bottle.

Don't comb relaxer through your hair—it'll lose elasticity and eventually break. Use your fingers, the back of a comb or even a tongue depressor to distribute the relaxer.

Use a timer. Don't leave a relaxer on your hair for longer than 25 minutes, and only coarse hair can tolerate it that long without breaking. As little as 10 to 15 minutes with a mild relaxer is usually enough to straighten fine kinky hair.

Rinse, rinse, rinse. Be sure no relaxer remains on your hair and scalp. Shampoo three times and rinse thoroughly again. Relaxer left on your hair will continue breaking it down and cause major damage.

Condition your hair. Apply a deep moisturizing and protein conditioner. Cover it with a plastic cap, then rinse after 20 minutes.

Don't relax and color your hair yourself. Wait at least two weeks before coloring your hair, and go to a professional for the safest results.

The Breaking Point

To overcome hairline breakage, you need a recovery plan. Here are some solutions to this very common concern.

BREAKAGE AT THE NAPE

Cause: Wool collars, hats and scarves may be the culprit here.

Rx: To camouflage, have the nape tapered, then start fresh and avoid the irritant. Cover your collars and line hats with silk or satin.

HAIRLINE BREAKAGE

Cause: Chemicals staying on the hair too long or curling irons that singe the hair can create breakage at the hairline. Braiding or pulling or setting hair tightly will weaken the hairline and cause it to recede.

Rx: Massage your temples and the rest of your hairline to stimulate circulation and bring blood to the area. This will encourage growth. Refrain from tight styles that put pressure on the hairline.

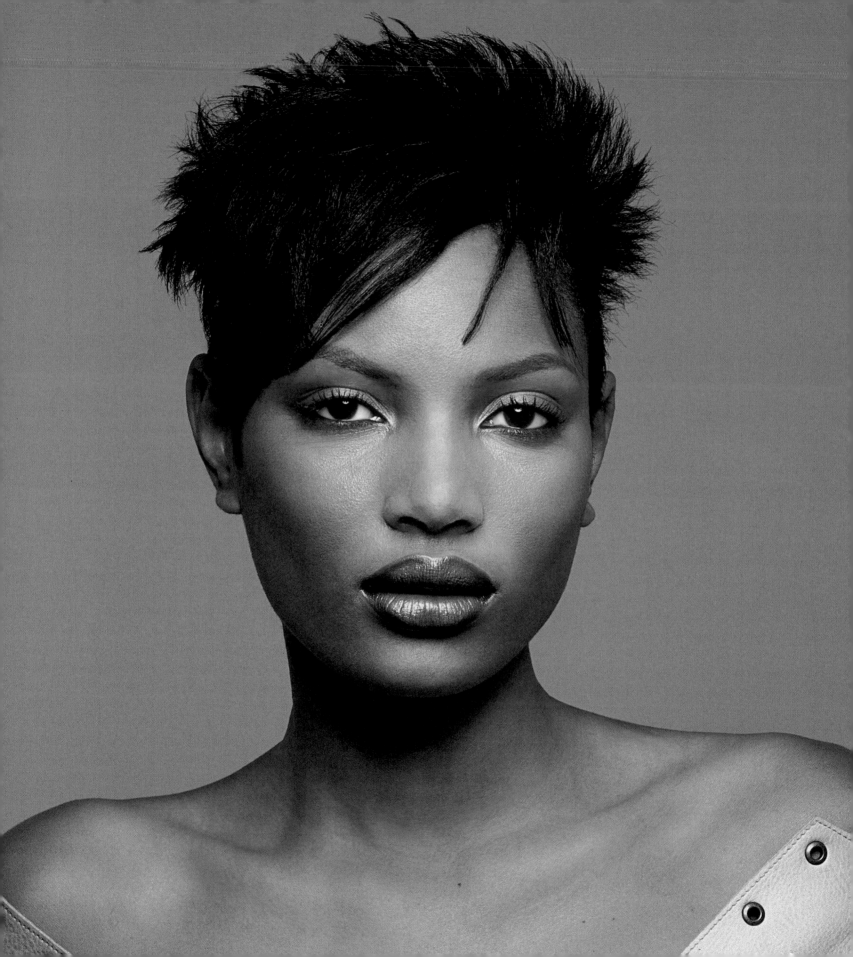

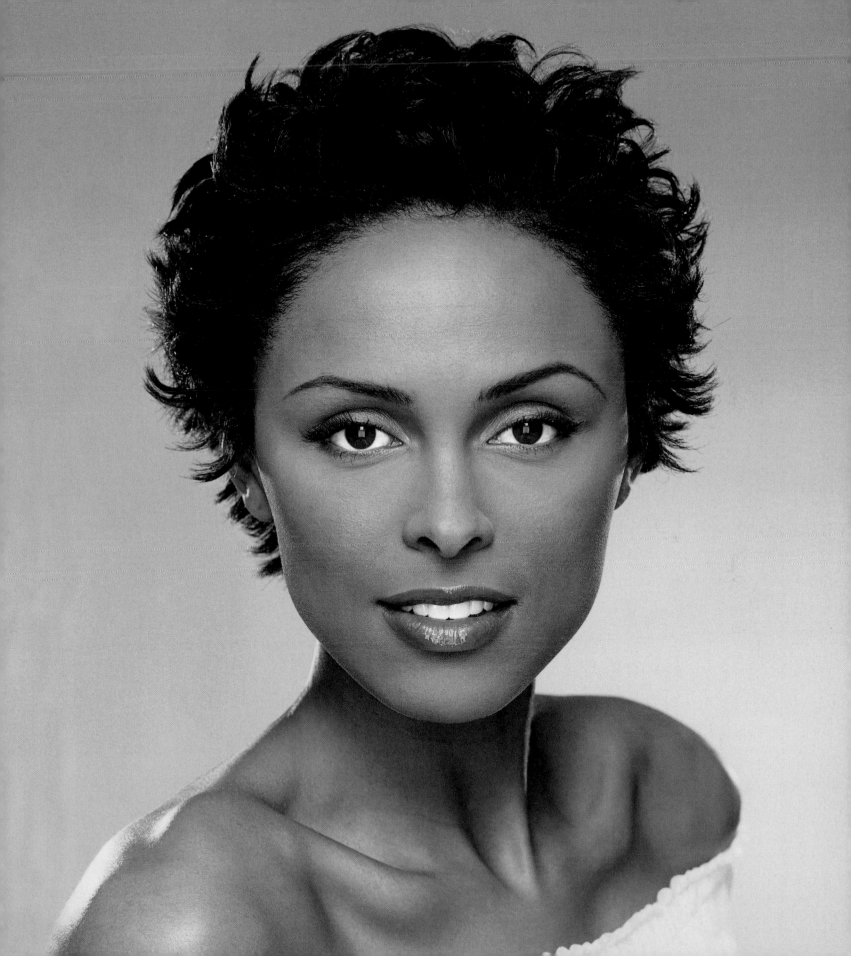

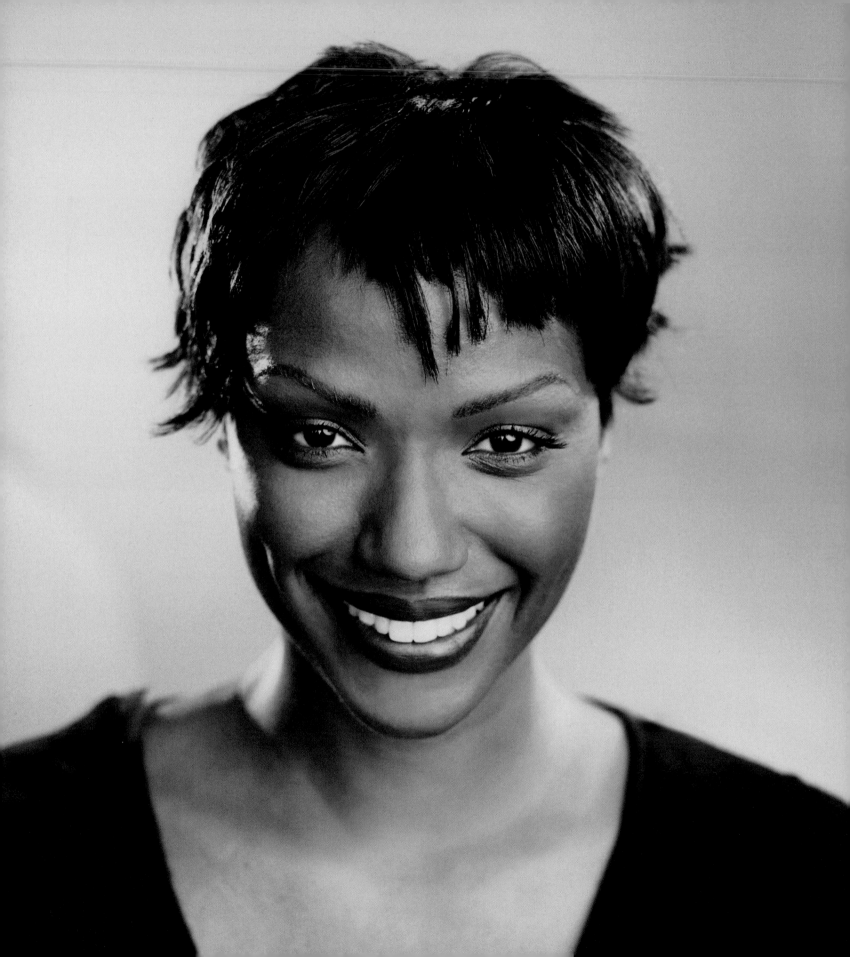

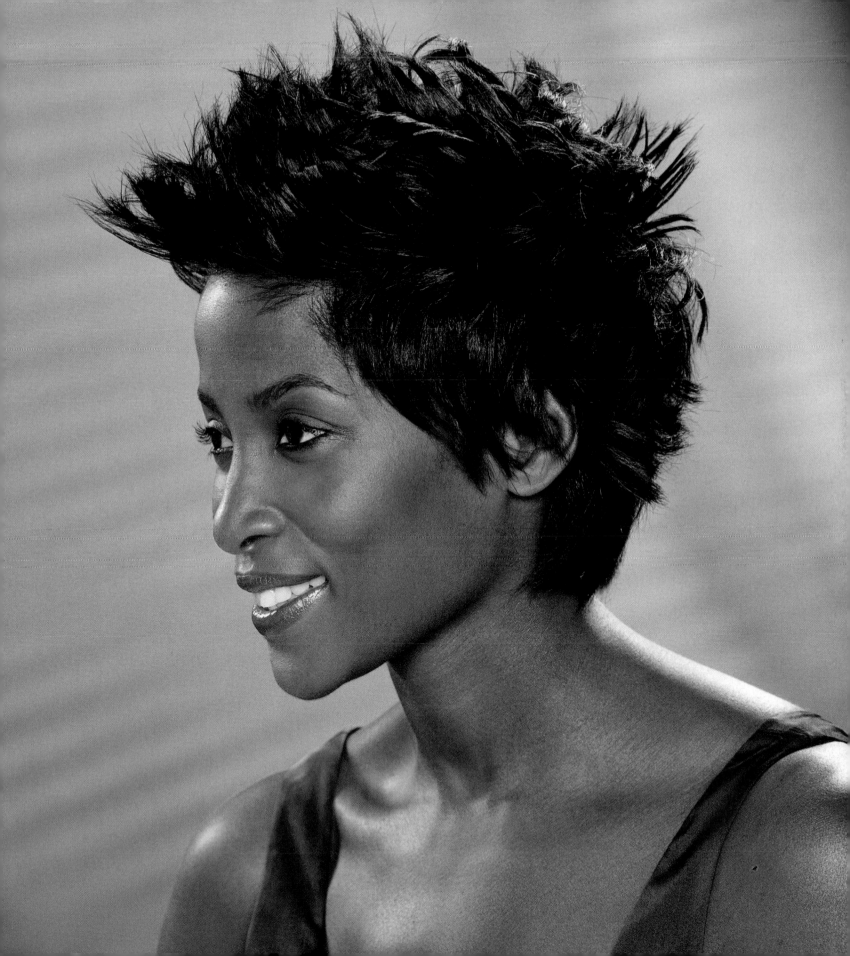

Thanks to a plethora of hair-care products for us, going from straight to textured-looking hair is easier than ever. Saturate freshly washed, soaking-wet hair with a setting lotion, then create two-strand twists and sit under a hooded dryer for 30 minutes. Once dry, remove and style with fingers.

The Transition: Going From Relaxed to Natural Hair

Sometimes your hair just needs a break from chemicals. Today more and more sisters are freeing themselves from endless touch-ups and damaging heated appliances. Many of us are going back to our natural hair texture and loving it! But seamlessly transitioning from straight to natural hair requires patience and effort. Years ago, the only choice available was to cut off all the hair and start with a short natural. Today's experts have found several ways to grow out of a relaxer and keep hair healthy and looking great.

Five Ways to Return to Your Roots

1. Roller Sets (instead of wrap-setting the hair)
Results: You'll get a head full of curls to hide the bulkiness of new growth.

2. Pressing or Flat-Ironing the New Growth
Results: Supercareful styling with heat will straighten kinky roots, but you have to be so careful to not apply the heat to the relaxed part of your hair shaft. This is critical to prevent breakage.

3. Braiding with Hair Extensions
Results: New growth is hidden with individual braids or cornrows, leaving the transitional process completely invisible.

4. Sewn-In Weave
Results: Your hair is cornrowed underneath and completely hidden, making the transition undetectable. Caution: The thread can cut into your own hair if it's sewn too tight.

5. Going Short
Results: Close-cropped looks are fashion-forward and look great. Get a beautiful, short precision cut.

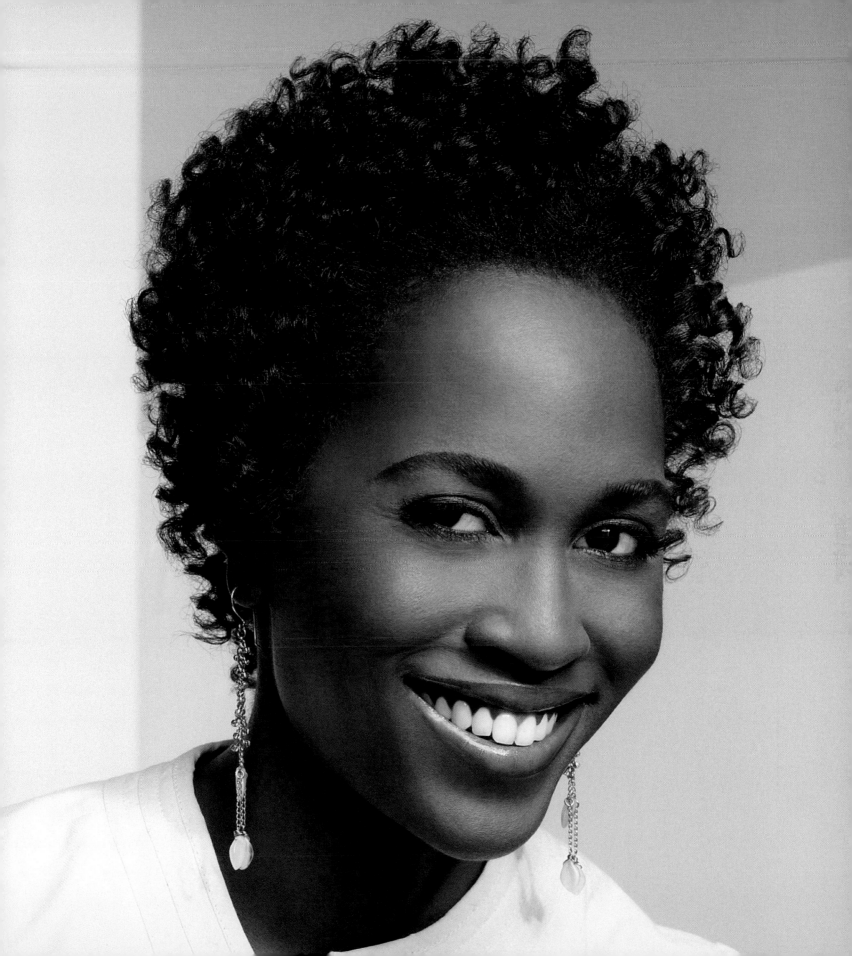

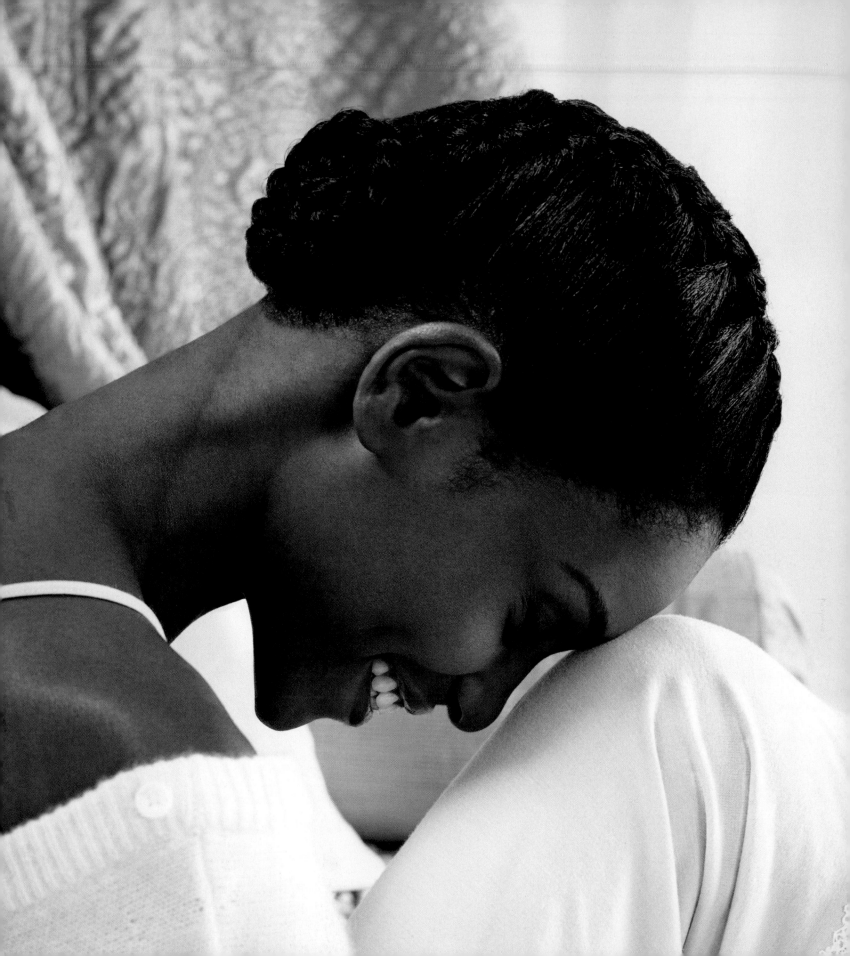

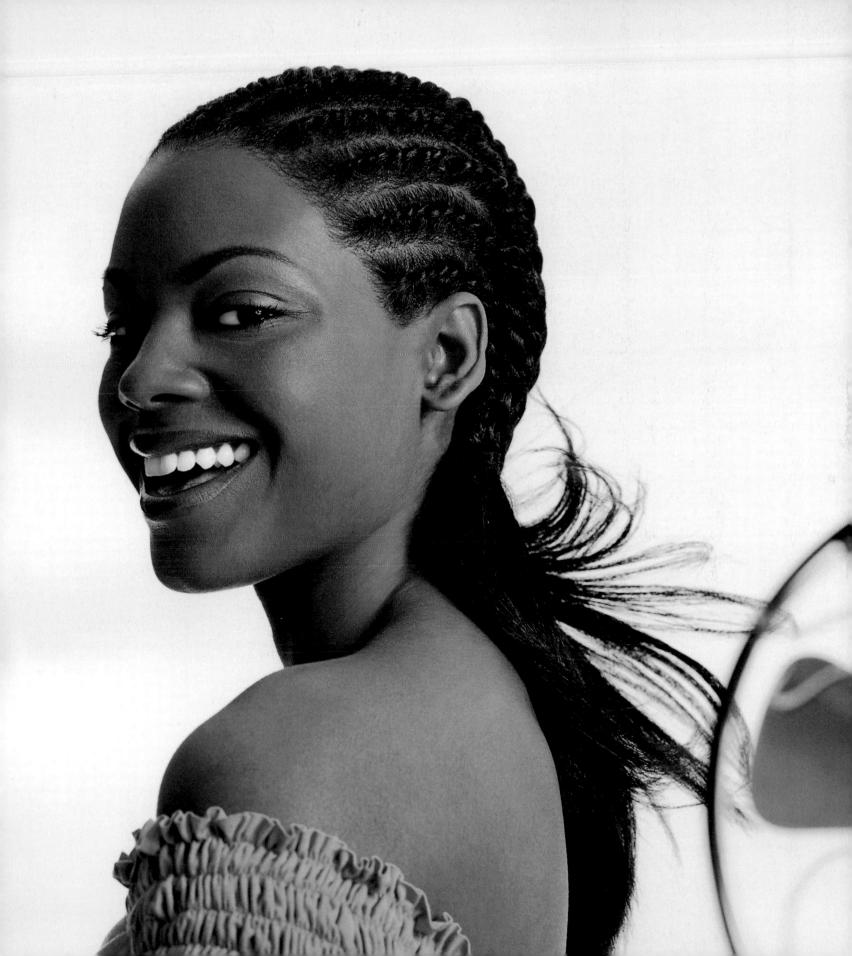

Natural Wonder: Caring for Your Natural Hair

More and more sisters are embracing the wondrous textures of their hair and celebrating its versatility with bodacious 'fros, beautiful braids, tempting twists and luxurious locks. But chemical-free hair isn't synonymous with fuss-free care. Our hair requires maintenance, whether it's processed or natural. Here's how to keep natural hair gorgeous.

➤ **Shampooing:** Wash your hair weekly with a moisturizing shampoo that has extra emollients. Those formulated for dry or damaged hair are most nourishing. Shampoo at least every two weeks if you sport braids and cornrows.

➤ **Conditioning:** Follow each shampoo with a rinse-out conditioner. Once a month give yourself a hot-oil treatment, which helps seal in moisture. Moisturize your hair daily with a light cream or natural oil, like jojoba or sweet almond. When wearing cornrows or individual braids, apply a light oil to your scalp once or twice a week.

➤ **Combing out:** There is a special way to handle natural tresses during the combing-out process. Whether your hair is wet or dry, first work in a moisturizing cream to soften it. Using a wide-toothed comb, detangle the hair from the ends going toward the roots.

➤ **Drying:** You can air-dry, hood-dry or blow-dry with a diffuser. If you want straighter hair, blow-dry in sections with a comb attachment.

➤ **Styling:** Just as with relaxed tresses, make sure to apply heat to clean hair that's been prepped with a dressing cream. Try to avoid extreme heat because it will diminish the hair's elasticity, causing breakage. To straighten and curl your natural, blow-dry, then use a hot comb and/or flat iron and curling iron.

Natural-Hair Time Line

DAY TO DAY

Massage the scalp. Take a few minutes each day to massage your scalp, with or without oil—even if you wear your hair braided or twisted. This simple practice stimulates the secretion of sebaceous oils and stimulates blood circulation.

Coddle at night. Take five minutes to pamper your hair before bedtime. That means moisturizing if necessary, securing the ends and covering at night.

WEEK TO WEEK

Moisturize. Most natural hair soaks up moisture like a sponge, so moisturize, moisturize, moisturize with natural oils.

Deep treat. After your weekly shampoo, take a few more minutes to condition your hair with deep treatments—especially during the winter months. Hot oil is good for stationary styles (like braids and twists); rich, creamy hair masks are great for loose, natural hair. Put on a plastic cap and let the conditioner sink in 10 to 15 minutes before you rinse.

MONTH TO MONTH

Steam treat. Steam treatments allow water and conditioners to deep-penetrate the hair shaft. First shampoo and rinse, apply your favorite deep treatment, then wrap your hair in a warm towel. Sit in a steamy bathroom for 20 to 30 minutes.

Get regular trims. Trim every four to six weeks to maintain your style and keep ends healthy or every six to eight weeks if you are growing your hair out.

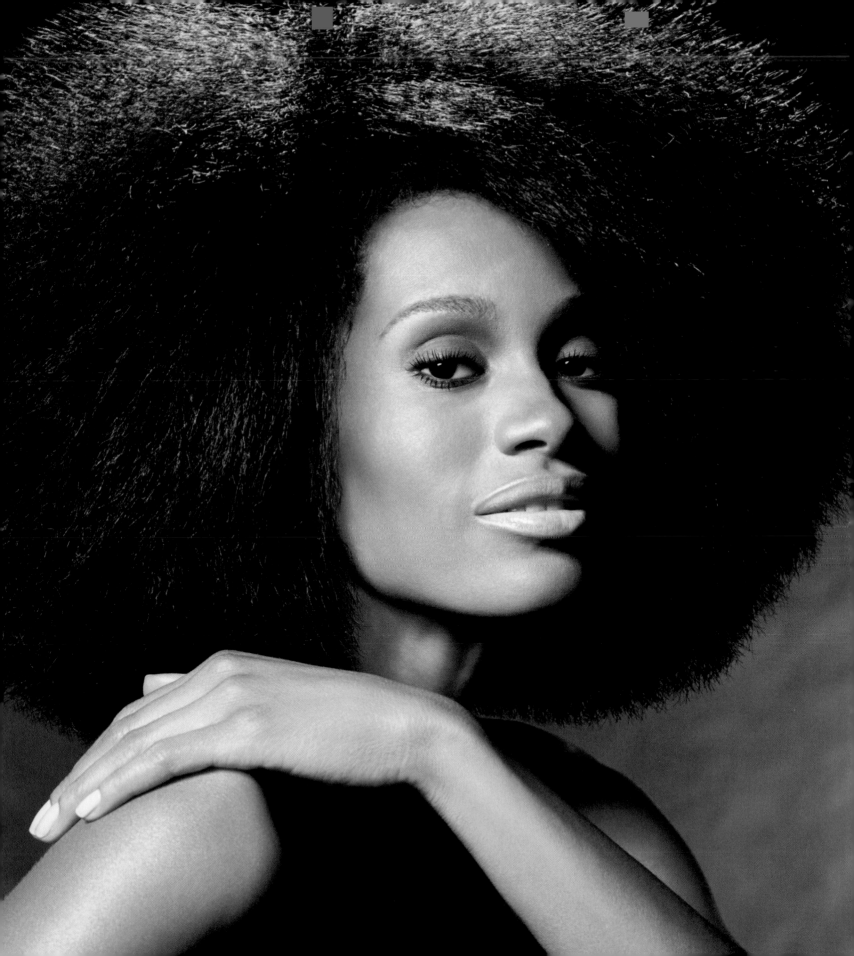

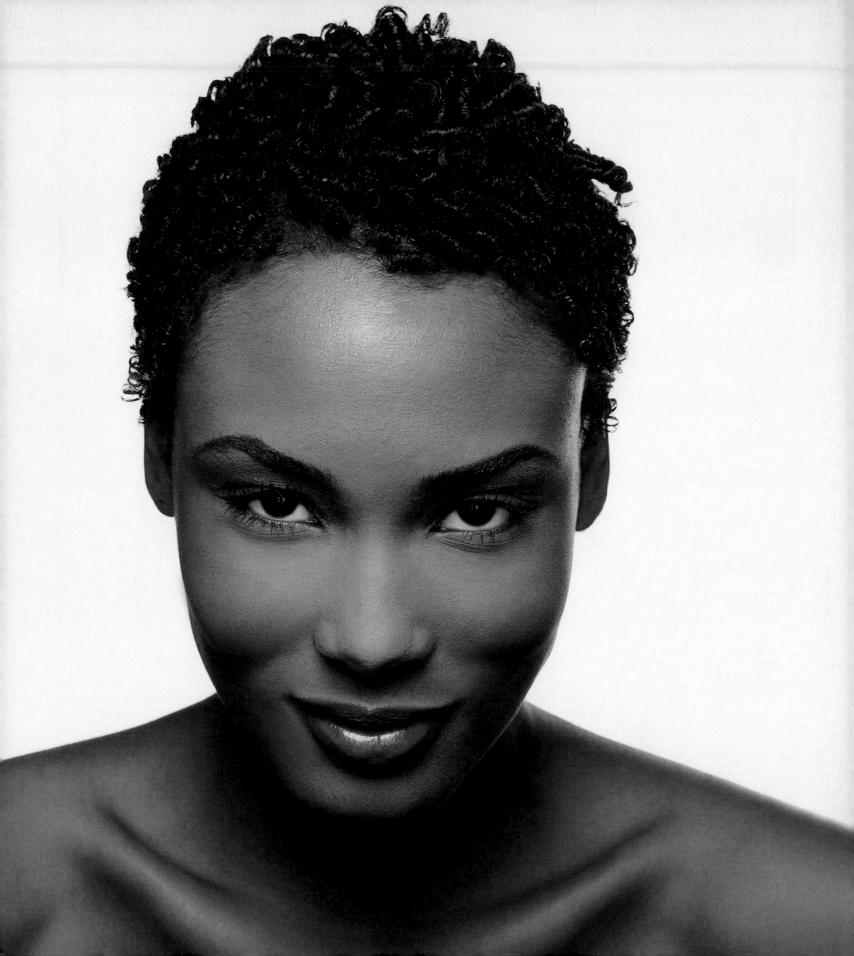

Braids and Twists

Braids have remained popular for decades because they give Black women a level of freedom we won't give up. Braided sisters work out, swim and sweat without worrying about their hair. And now, braids are more *in* than ever.

Individual Braids

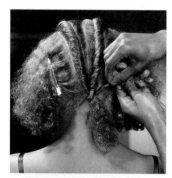

Maintenance: Wash your hair every week to ten days. If you're braiding with synthetic extensions, hair can be shampooed and conditioned as normal, but don't use creamy conditioners because they cause synthetic hair to slip and unravel. Braiding with human-hair extensions requires a lot more care. Before washing, you should braid together small handfuls of braids from the scalp to the ends and secure these larger braids at the end with covered bands. In the shower, shampoo and rinse the back of your hair, then tie on the sheerest scarf (one that water penetrates easily) and shampoo the front and sides. Don't rub vigorously. Gently press the shampoo onto your scalp and braids. Keep pressing the scalp and squeezing braids. Rinse and repeat twice more, keeping the scarf in place. Condition and rinse well. Then remove the scarf for a final rinse. Lower the water pressure a bit to prevent extensions from slipping. Pressing a hand-held shower head lightly over your scalp is the best way to ensure your hair is thoroughly rinsed. But do keep your scarf on so braids stay beautiful. Be sure not to leave any residue of shampoo or conditioner on your scalp. Smooth on a leave-in conditioner and a light alcohol-free gel; then tie your hair flat with a scarf. Every two to three days, moisturize the scalp with lightweight natural hair oils. Spray-on is a good choice. Cover with a scarf or stocking cap before bed.

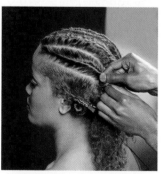

Duration: Individual braids can last up to three months. Between braidings, have your hairline and any braids that have gotten fuzzy rebraided. With braids kept in longer, your hair will begin to lock.

Two-Strand Twists

Maintenance: Usually, the ends are braided, tied with holders (for a child) or set on rollers to keep them from unraveling. Shampoo at least every two weeks and retwist. Apply a lightweight oil to the scalp once a week, and cover with a scarf or stocking cap before bed.

Duration: Twists last up to two weeks. Note: If you want a gorgeous, full and wavy natural look, untwist your hair after drying and lightly finger-comb.

Cornrows

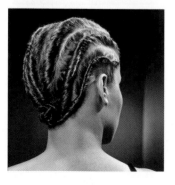

Maintenance: Lubricate the scalp with lightweight oils. To keep the edges flat, each morning smooth on a dab of nonalcohol gel, tie on a scarf and dry for a few seconds with a blower. See "Braids" for information on shampooing and drying your hair.

Duration: Cornrows last up to one month. If they're kept in longer, your hair will look fuzzy.

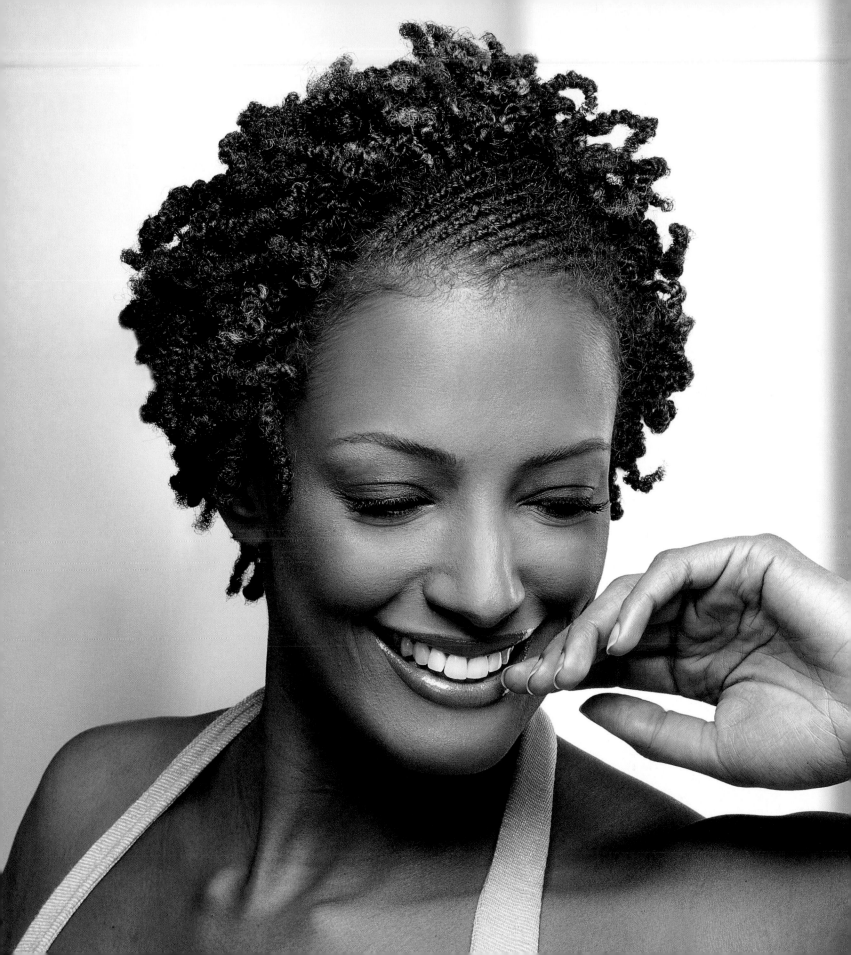

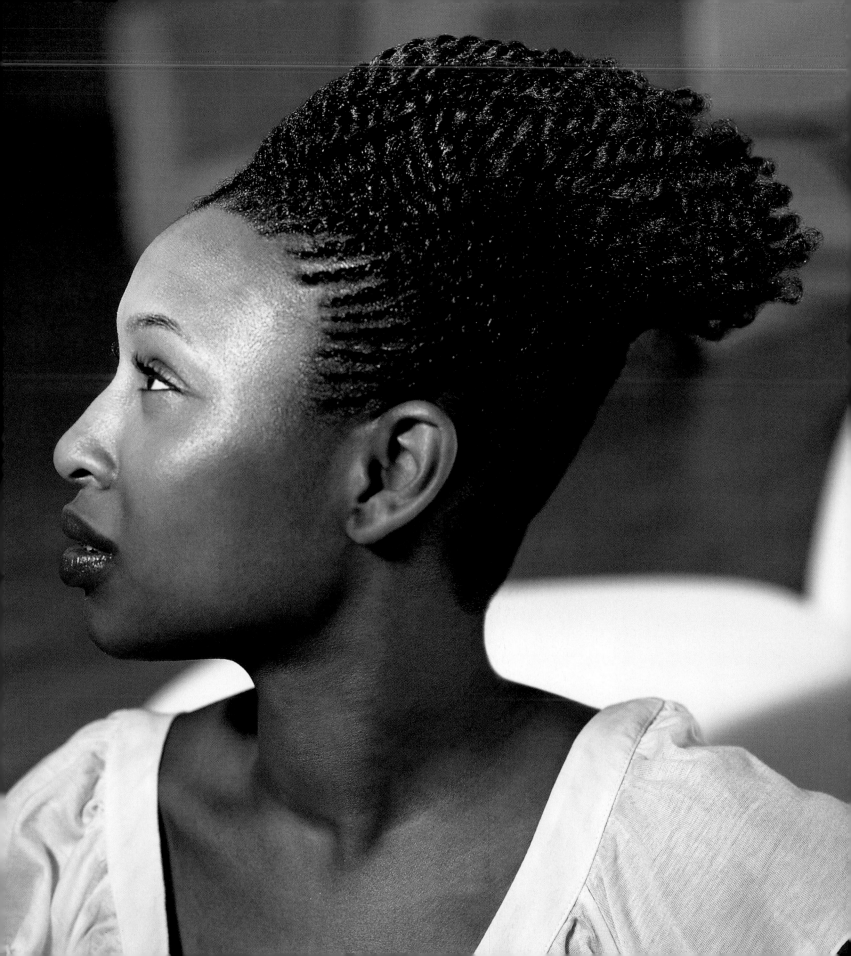

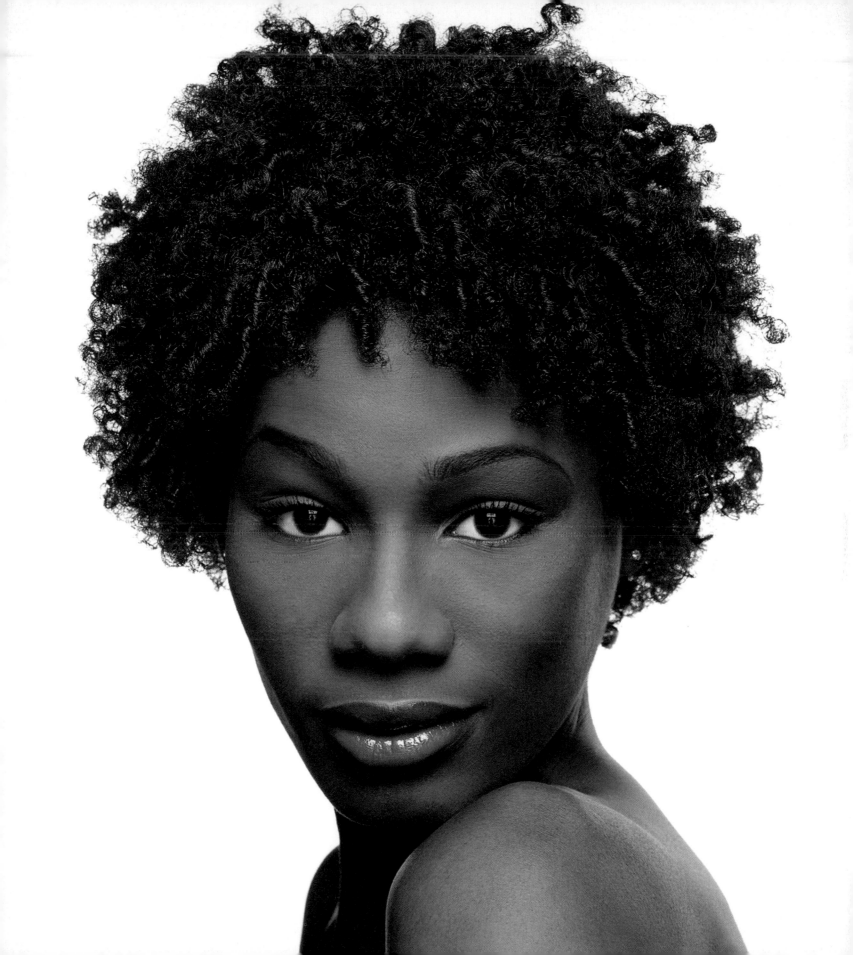

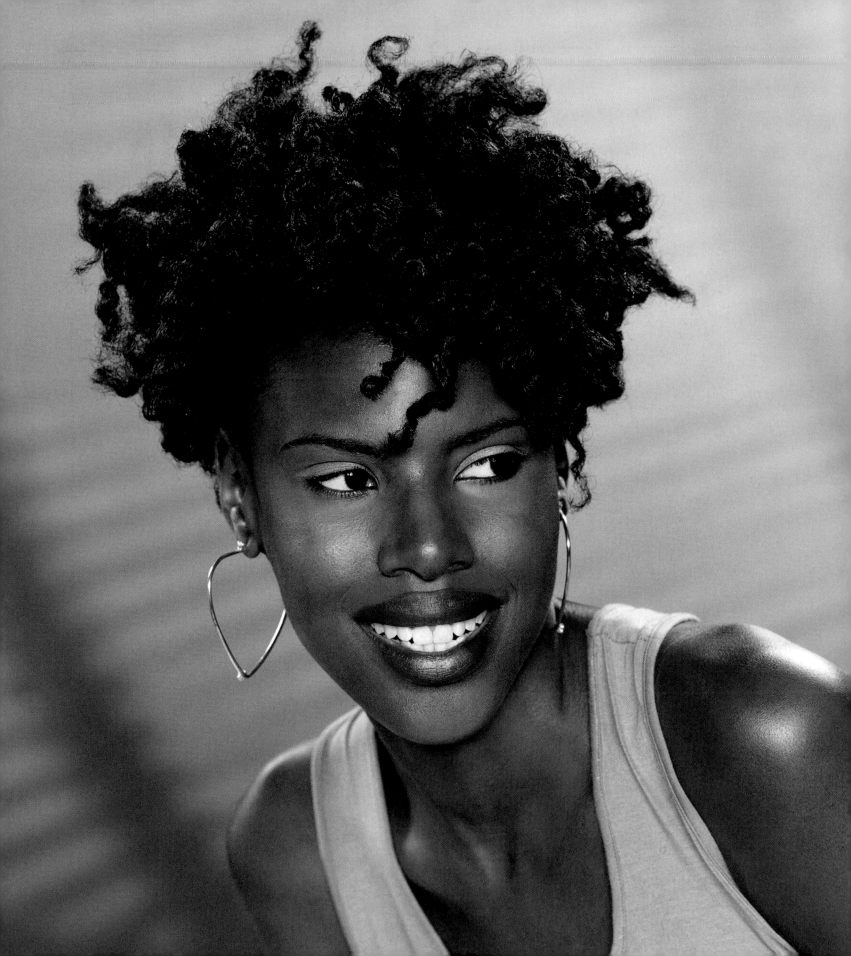

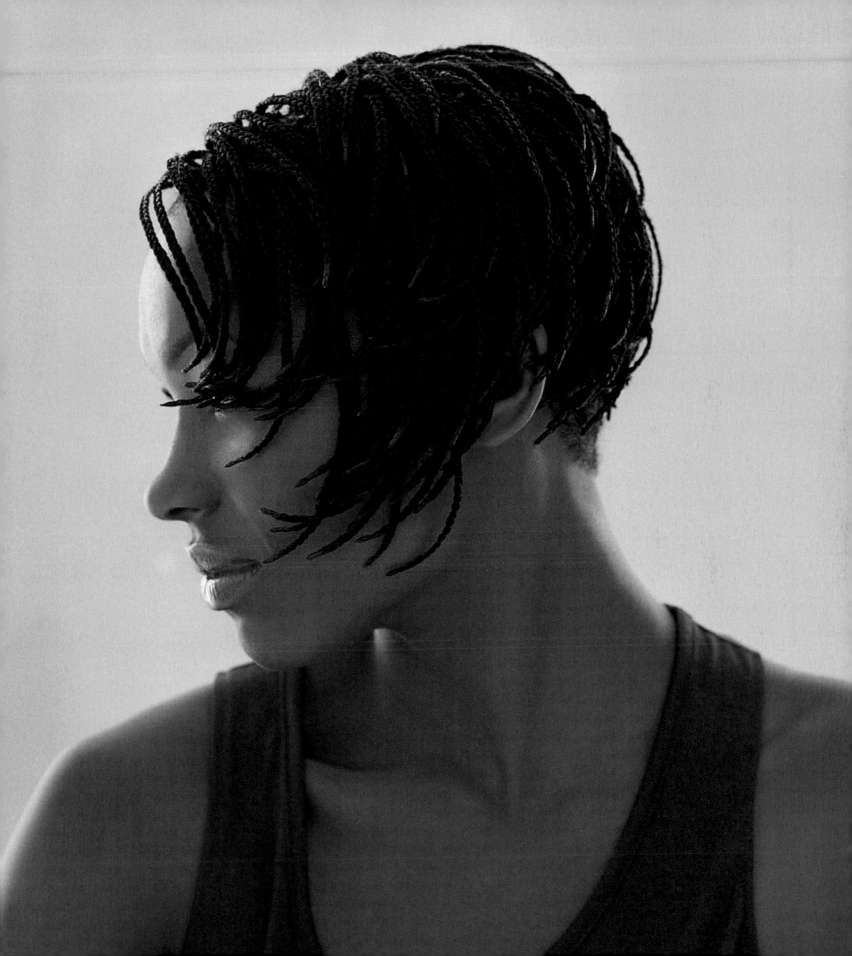

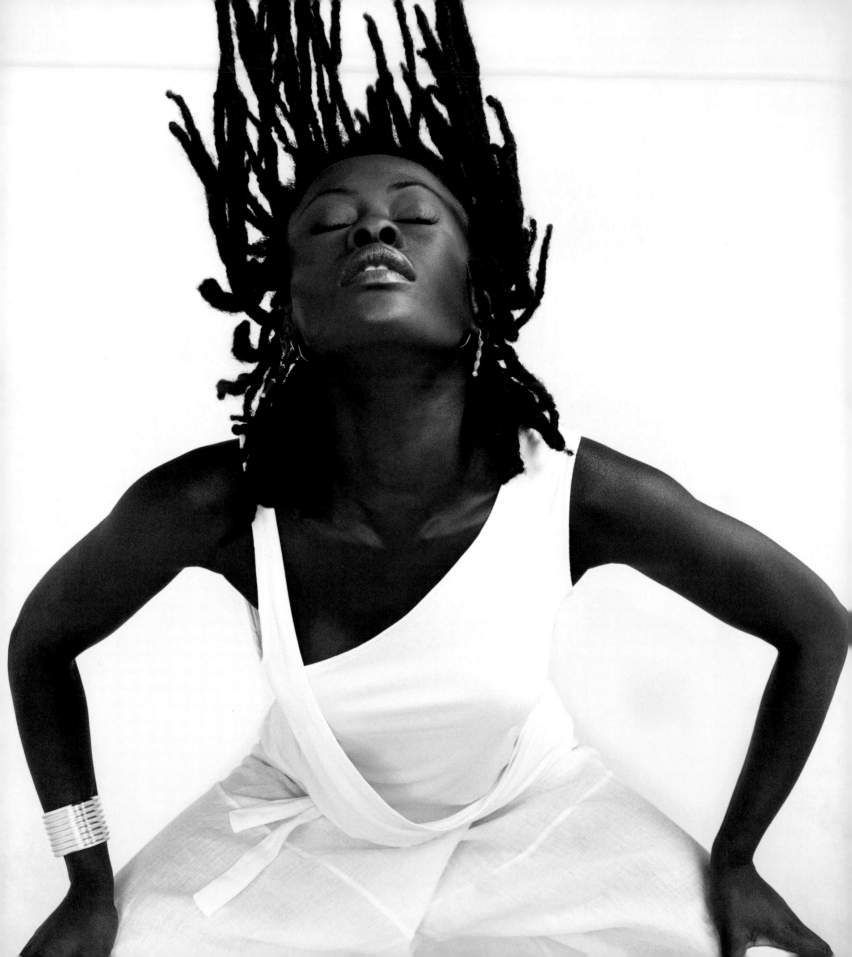

Caution: Never allow anyone to braid your or your child's hair so tightly that it hurts. This technique will eventually cause permanent hair loss. Styles that fall forward put much less stress on the hairline.

Caring for Braids

To fully enjoy your braided look, remember these tips:

➤ **Shampoo** and condition frequently, every week to ten days.
➤ **Avoid** creamy conditioners, which can leave a noticeable buildup and cause extensions to slip and unbraid. Stick to lightweight leave-in conditioners.
➤ **Use** styling glaze or gel to tame frizzies and to smooth the hairline.
➤ **Try** a spray-on oil sheen to help keep braids looking fresh.
➤ **Cover** your braids at night with a scarf or stocking cap.

Lock Star

More frequently than ever, sisters are choosing to wear locks, a healthy and gorgeous choice for our hair. Locks make a powerful statement about racial pride and our natural beauty. Many sisters and brothers who wear locks feel their hair is sacred. The style gets its name from the "locking" process that occurs when hair is not combed, brushed or manipulated—causing strands to intertwine permanently.

Locticians, hairstylists who specialize in creating and maintaining locks, have devised several techniques to achieve polished, fabulous-looking locks—which are growing in popularity among both women and men. Here are three ways to create locks.

Hand Coil

How It's Done: Divide the hair into small sections. Then, working a water-soluble gel into the hair, twirl each section between your index finger and thumb to form a lock. Twirl to the strand's end.

Time Frame for Results: The difficult part is in the beginning: You can't wash your hair vigorously until it begins to lock together, which can take six to eight weeks, depending on the texture of your hair. The more coily and thick your hair is, the faster it will lock.

Maintenance: Until you are able to shampoo thoroughly, cleanse your scalp with a cotton swab dipped in antiseptic, spray your scalp with a mixture of water and antiseptic, or wash hair gently wearing a stocking cap.

Palm Roll

How It's Done: Roll small, parted sections of natural hair between both palms with a water-soluble gel to create coils.

Time Frame for Results: You'll have locks in about six weeks.

Maintenance: Do not shampoo or condition locks vigorously during the first six weeks; or simply cleanse with an antiseptic and lubricate the scalp.

For a crinkle set, wash and condition locks, then braid them with smaller, tighter plaits toward the front. After locks dry, which usually takes 24 hours, unbraid them. The style will last from shampoo to shampoo. You only need a touch of moisturizing oil and some finger styling.

Faux Locks: Lock Extensions

How It's Done: Sections of matted or locked human hair are sewn, braided or looped with a crochet needle into your hair to achieve a "locked" look.

Time Frame for Results: This technique requires 12 to 18 hours—but once it's done, you'll never have to remove the extensions or redo the process. Overnight, you can have gorgeous locks of any length you choose.

Maintenance: You can shampoo and condition your hair as normal. Retwist hair every four to six weeks.

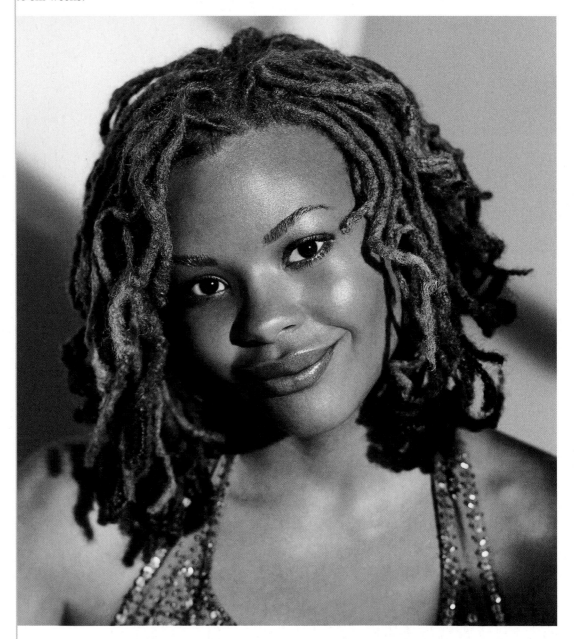

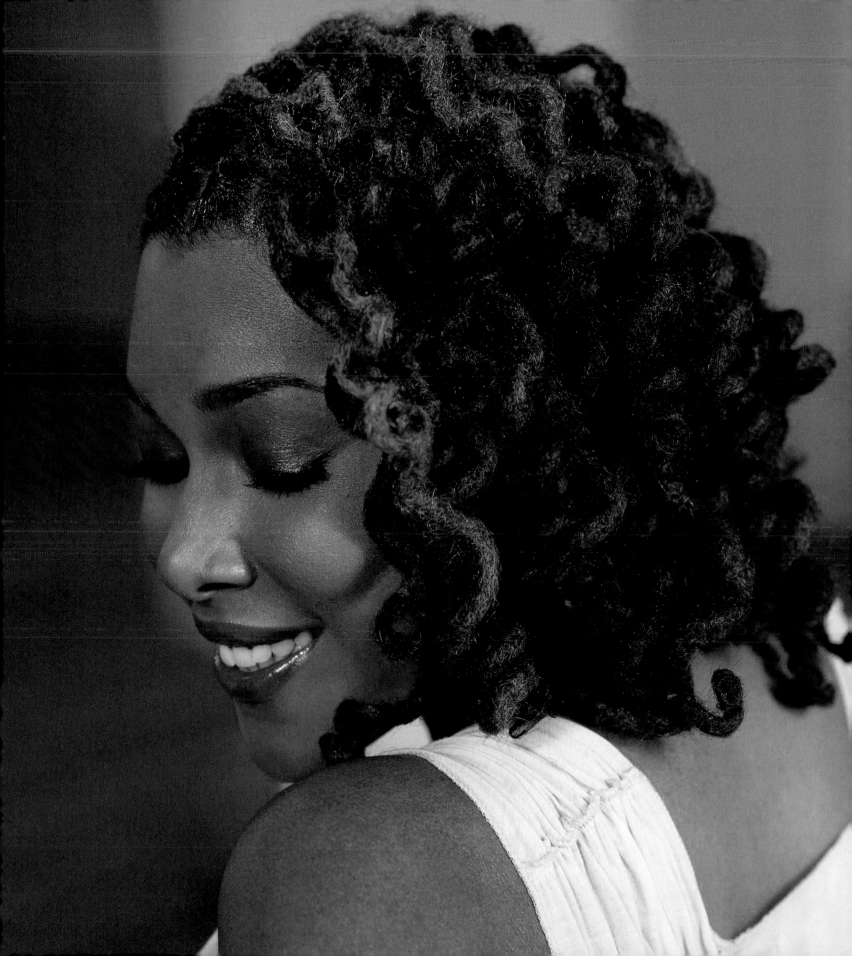

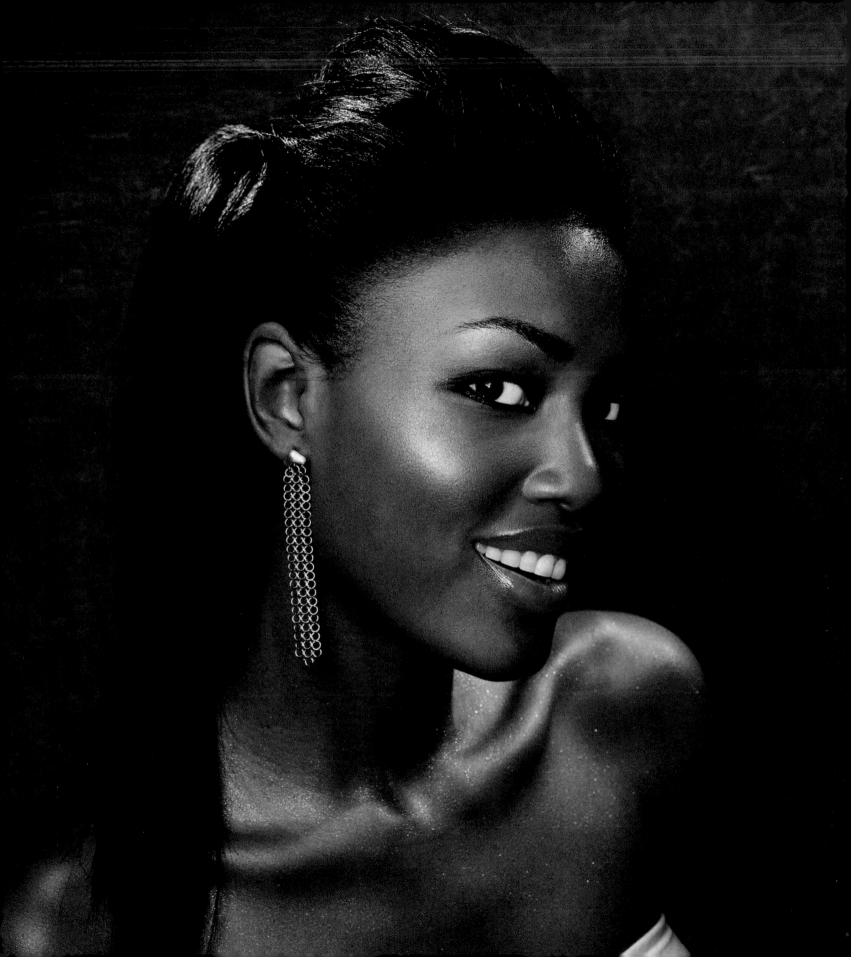

Hair Extending

We women love options, and extending our hair is a quick way to create a new look. Here's a brief guide to methods that can change your length and style in a few hours.

Bonding

How It's Done: Wefts of hair are glued to the shaft of your hair close to the scalp.

Pros: This approach is quick. It takes only a few minutes to apply each weft, which can add volume and length.

Cons: The glue can cause skin irritation and infection, and improper removal can cause hair breakage. We recommend skipping this option.

Sewing

How It's Done: First your hair is cornrowed, then wefts of hair are sewn onto your cornrowed hair.

Pro: This method gives your hair a rest and won't irritate your scalp.

Cons: Great care must be taken when removing the weave. You risk damaging your hair along the shaft when cutting out the stitches or if the thread is too tight.

Interlocking

How It's Done: This is a variation of the sewing technique—but without the cornrows. A microthin weft is sewn onto your loose hair.

Pro: Because there are no cornrows, the weave is flat in appearance, allowing for a more natural look and feel.

Con: The weft and sewing may become undone if hair is brushed too vigorously.

Strand by Strand

How It's Done: Your hair is divided into small sections, each braided an inch or more with extensions, then sewn or wrapped with thread to secure it.

Pros: This braiding method is a healthier application than gluing. It lasts from six to ten weeks, depending on how fast your hair grows out.

Con: Because hair is braided near the scalp, parted styles aren't easily achieved.

Fusion

How It's Done: Strands of human hair are attached to sections of your own hair with a keratin-protein bond or wax that matches your hair color.

Pros: This technique offers lots of versatility, and you can run your fingers through your hair.

Con: You must be supergentle, or your hair will unbond. Removal can cause damage if specifically designed fusion remover is not used.

Weave-Care Time Line

DAY TO DAY

Feed your hair and scalp. Moisturize and condition your weave and your scalp with light, natural oil. This regimen will feed your scalp and lessen the shedding that occurs when the extensions are removed.

Maintain the curl pattern. Give your wavy or curly-textured extensions a daily spritz of water and leave-in conditioner to keep the curl pattern uniform.

WEEK TO WEEK

Shampoo weekly. Weaves need to be cleansed frequently to look fresh.

Keep it dry. If your hair is cornrowed, bacteria and mildew can grow on your scalp and hair if they remain damp for a long time. Make sure that your hair is completely dry after you shower, shampoo or swim.

MONTH TO MONTH

Moisturize before you remove your hair. This treatment will help cut back on shedding.

Keep it up. See your stylist every three to four weeks so he or she can groom and refresh your extensions.

Be timely. Never leave extensions in for more than three months. They will lock at the base if left in longer.

Weave Know-How

Keep these pointers in mind when you're opting for a weave:

➤ Choose human hair or synthetic hair that can take heat.

➤ The better the quality of hair, the more natural it will look. It will probably be more expensive too.

➤ Consult with your hairstylist before purchasing the hair. He or she may have a specific place to recommend where you can purchase top-quality hair.

➤ Less is best when it comes to the amount of hair used. Many women make the mistake of adding too much hair.

➤ Select lightweight and microthin wefts. The thinner the weft, the less bulky the weave will look and feel.

➤ Match your hair with the purchased hair by mimicking the shade in the middle and ends of your hair; don't try to match the roots, which are usually darker.

➤ Don't weigh down a weave with heavy products like gels or moisturizing lotions. Instead, use light hair sprays with conditioners and sunscreen.

➤ Don't wait longer than three months to remove and redo a weave.

➤ Shampoo and condition your hair every week, just as you would if you weren't wearing a weave. Debris can easily find a resting place in weaves.

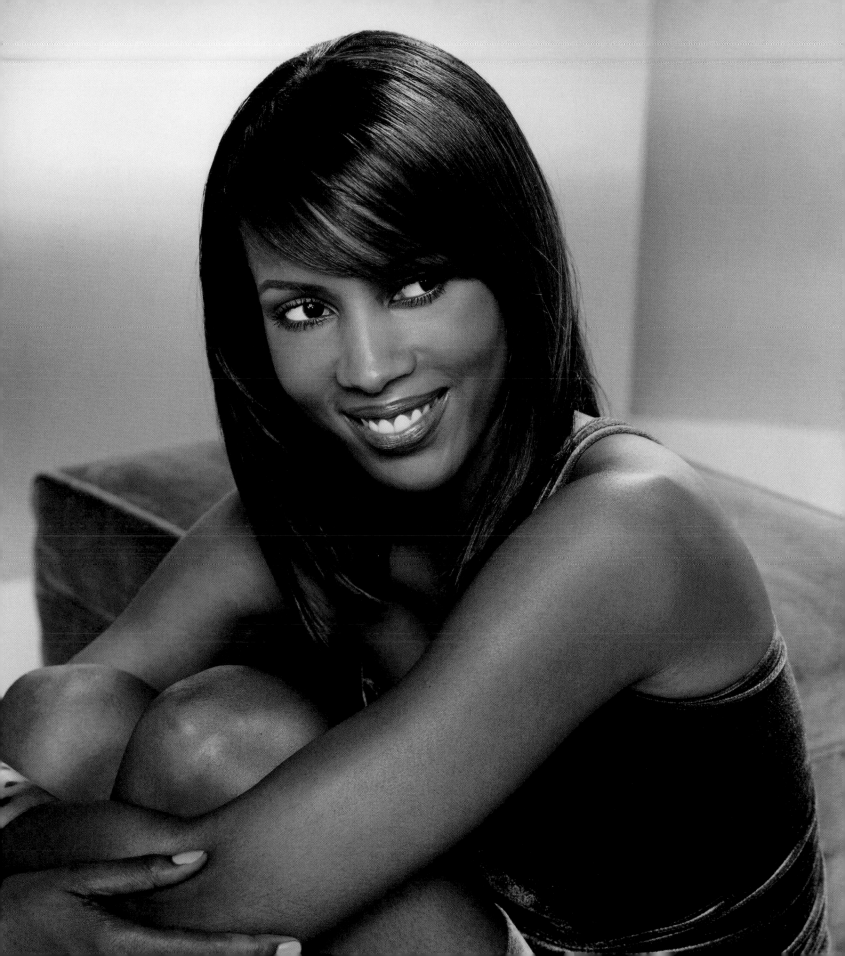

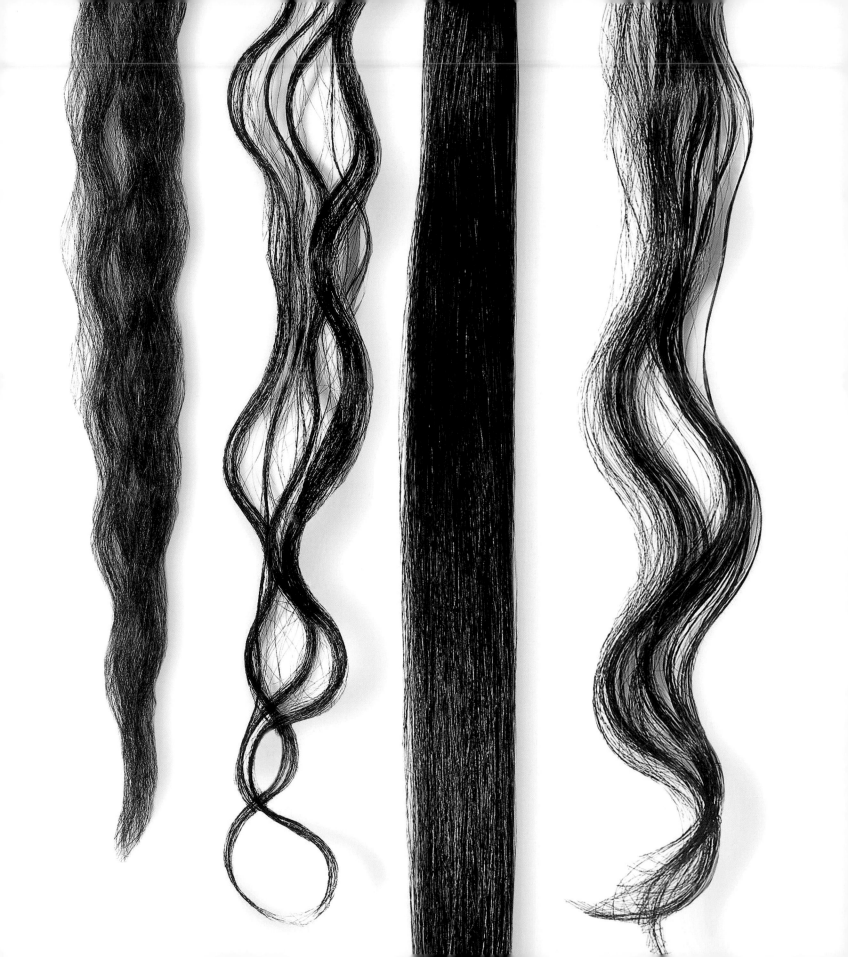

Wigging Out

Another way to change your look or just give your own hair a rest is to work a wig. Years ago, synthetic wigs didn't offer much in terms of styling options. But with the rise of custom-blended human-hair wigs, today we have many options offering short, midlength and longer styles that come highlighted, texturized, straight, wavy or curly—any way you want it. Here's a quick primer on wigs.

Custom Human Hair

Pro: You can change the style from straight to curly and anything in between.
Con: These wigs can be very expensive, up to thousands of dollars.

Synthetic Hair

Pro: These types of wigs offer an inexpensive way to get a new fabulous look.
Con: What you see is what you get. You can always cut the hair, but it's prestyled, so you cannot change it much or style with heated appliances. Note: There are now some synthetic fibers that can be styled with heat. Ask for synthetic wigs that offer that option.

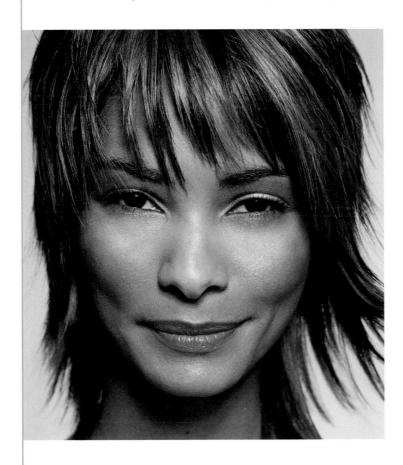

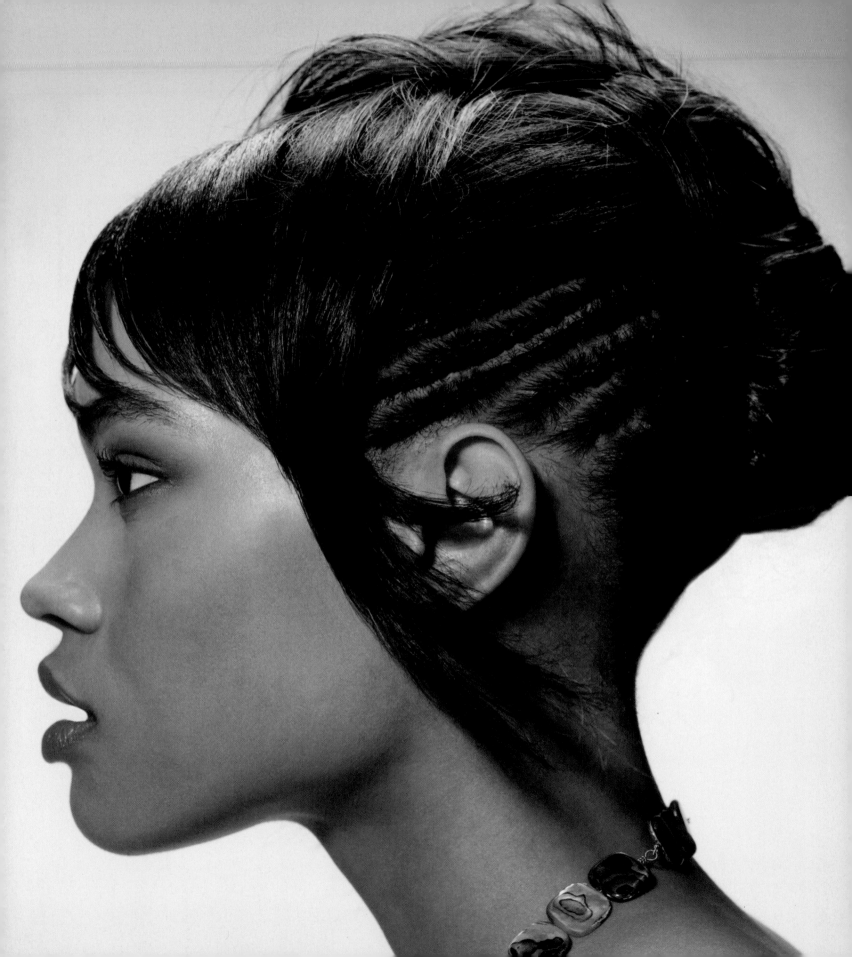

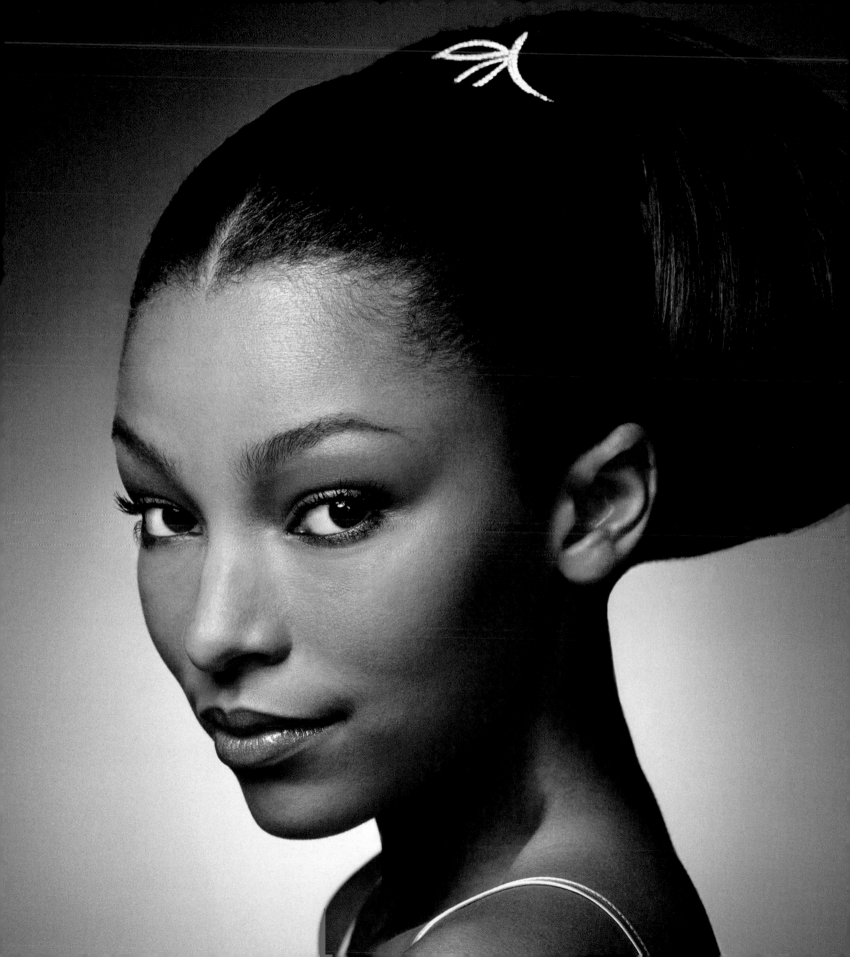

Coloring Your Hair

Some sisters are pulling out the stops: We're going platinum and golden and every shade of bronze. And now, formulations are safer and gentler than ever. Dyes are powerful chemicals, so if you can afford it, leave permanently coloring your hair to a pro. Here's the lowdown on common formulations and methods.

Hair-Coloring Formulas

Temporary Rinse

How It Works: The rinse is applied to the shaft to enhance your natural color.

Pros: A temporary rinse is gentle enough to apply on relaxed hair without damage. You can also use it at home.

Con: It only lasts from shampoo to shampoo.

Semipermanent

How It Works: A color formula, created without peroxide or ammonia, coats the hair shaft.

Pros: A semipermanent formula enriches your natural shade, covers gray and causes no damage.

Cons: It lasts only four to eight shampoos. And since the color doesn't penetrate the hair shaft, it cannot lighten but only darken hair.

Basic Color-Care Time Line

DAY TO DAY

Coat and protect. The sun can damage color-treated hair, so protect it from UVA and UVB rays with moisturizing hair products that contain sunscreen.

Think mild manipulation. The less you manipulate your hair with heated appliances, the better.

WEEK TO WEEK

Pick the best products. Styling aids designed for color-treated hair are formulated to help keep your color looking fresh and prevent fading.

Deep condition. After your weekly shampoo, always deep condition and add a leave-in conditioner just before you dry your hair.

MONTH TO MONTH

Choose chemical synergy. Try to leave three weeks between relaxing and permanently coloring your hair.

Keep pros in the know. If more than one person is giving you chemical treatments, it's important for each to know the formulations the other is using to ensure that they are complementary. And remember, nothing can damage your hair and create breakage faster than dual processes done incorrectly, so if you opt for both relaxing and permanent color, find the best-trained and highly recommended professionals.

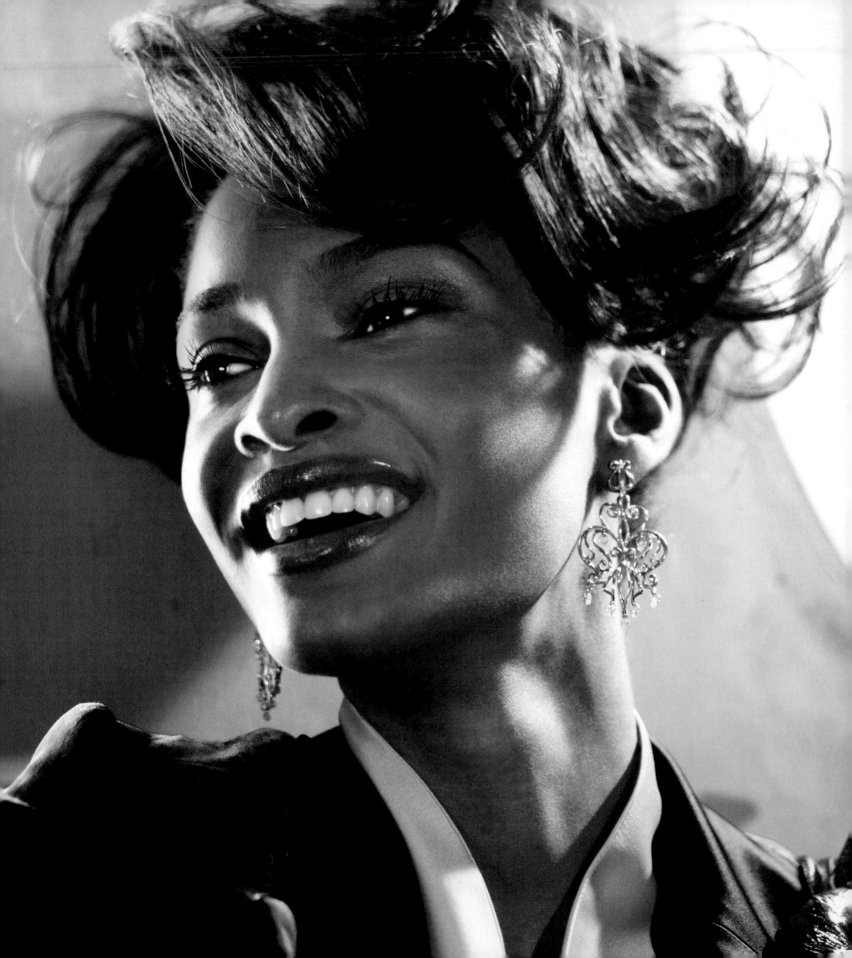

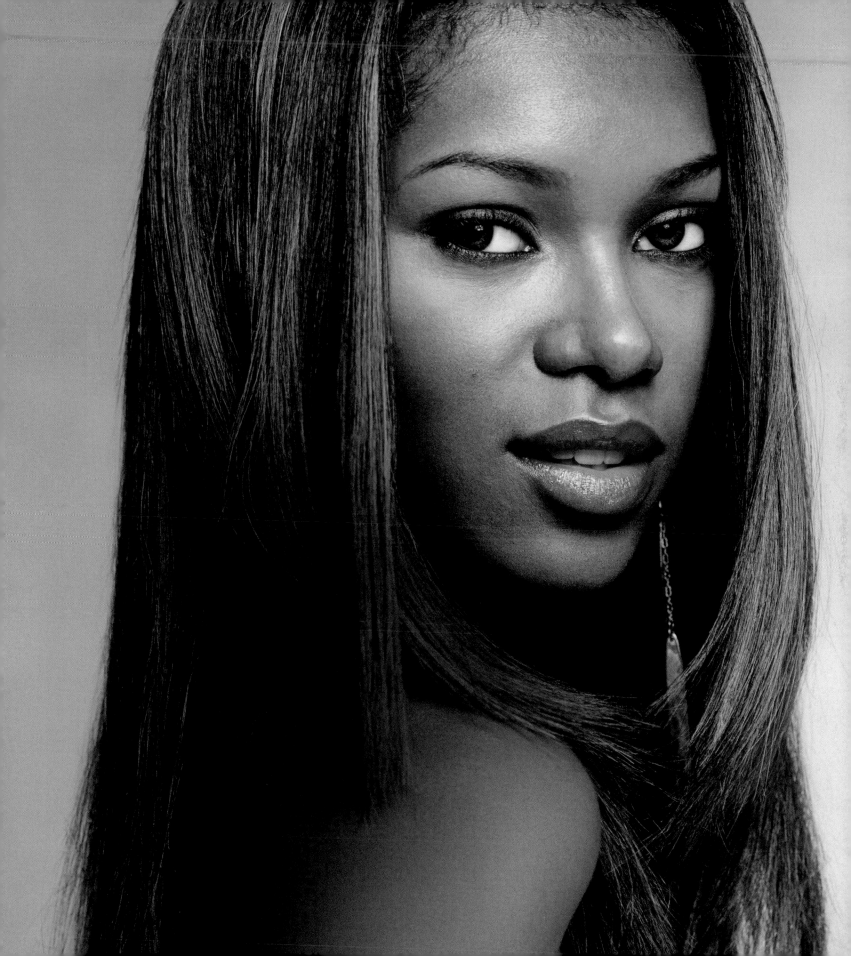

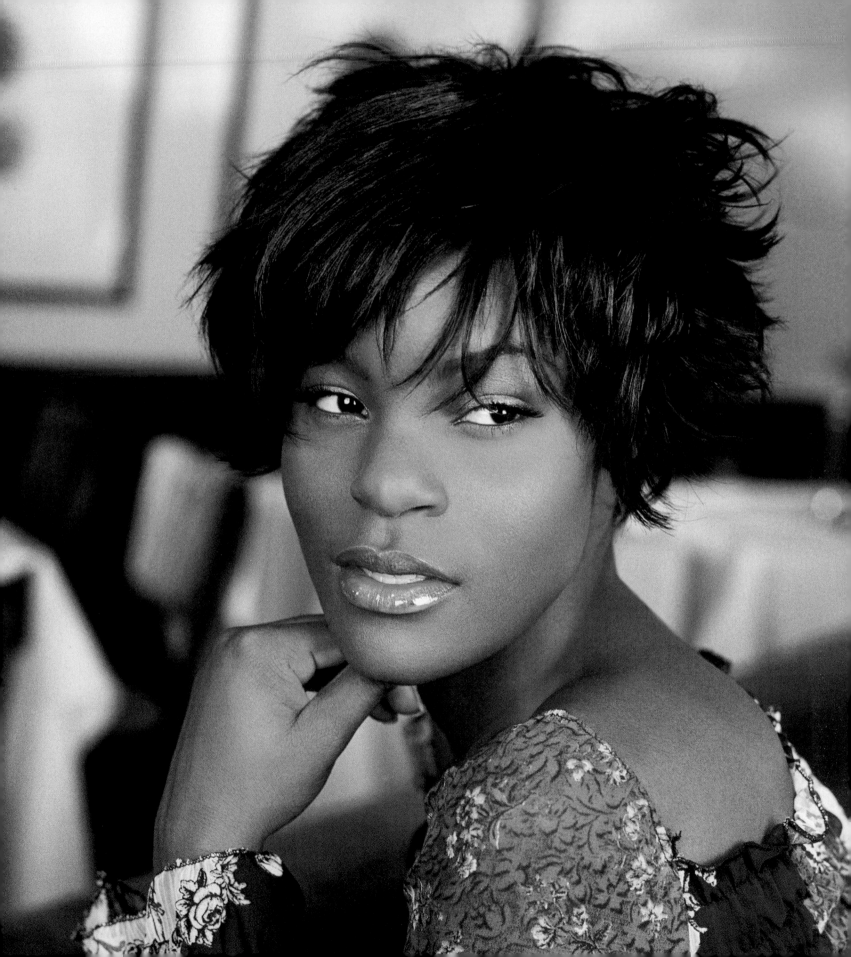

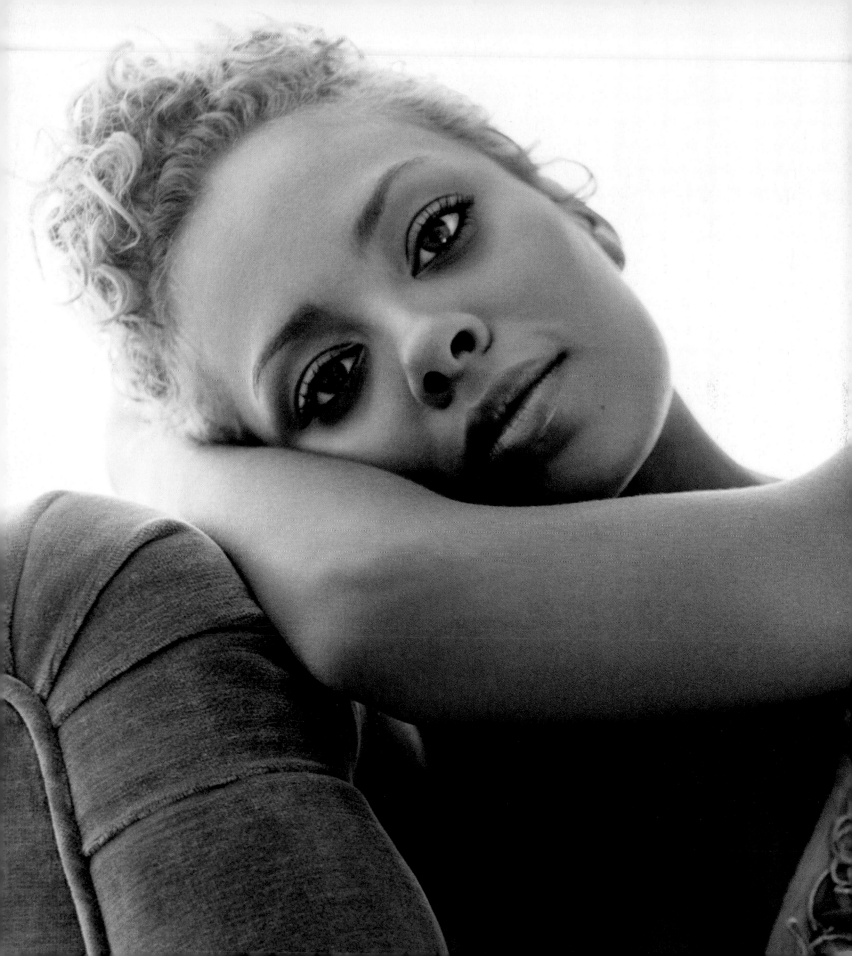

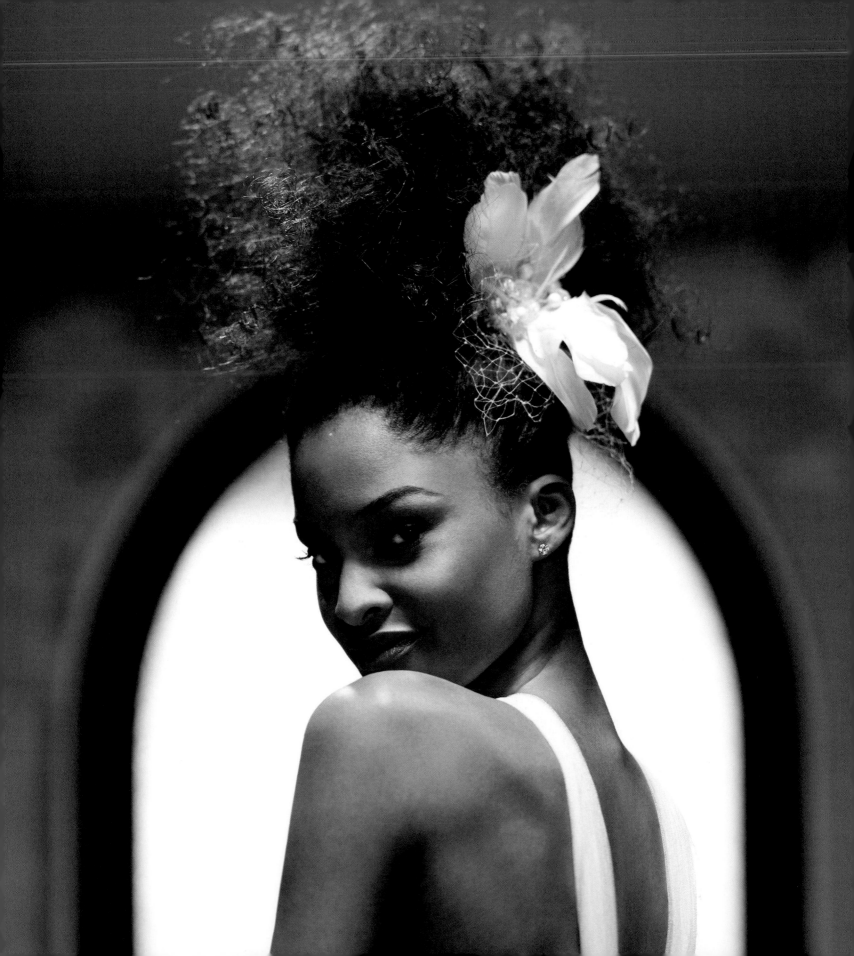

Steer clear of products with petroleum, which creates excessive buildup. And products with alcohol can strip hair of natural oils.

If your hair gets frizzy in humid weather, smooth your strands with a silicone-based gloss serum to seal the hair shaft, then use hot rollers to keep your curl.

Treat your scalp with nourishing oils between shampoos to protect against salt deposits from perspiration. These oils can also prevent irritation of the scalp from chemical processes, so apply the night before a chemical treatment.

Coloring at Home

Remember these do's and don't's for at-home coloring:

➤ Read the instructions thoroughly. Make sure you understand the entire coloring process before you begin. Follow the directions in the coloring kit precisely.
➤ Have everything you need laid out—gloves, applicator, towel—before starting. Once you apply color, you're on the clock. Don't get stuck without the necessary tools.
➤ Do a strand test. Test your skin 48 hours before coloring your hair to ensure you aren't allergic to the chemicals. If it's safe to proceed, take a small section of hair from the back of your head and apply the color formula. This way you'll know the result before you go all the way.

Demipermanent

How It Works: A formula consisting of pigment mixed with a low-grade peroxide (5 to 10 percent) deposits color onto the hair shaft.

Pros: It uses no ammonia, which can cause hair to dry out. It deepens and intensifies your existing color.

Con: You might need to wait at least two weeks after a relaxer to apply, depending on the condition of your hair.

Permanent

How It Works: Color is mixed with peroxide and ammonia to penetrate the hair shaft, which changes the hair's natural shade.

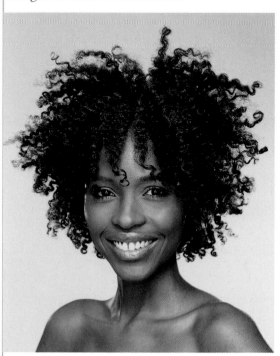

Pro: Permanent formulas can create a completely different color that cannot be rinsed away.

Cons: This type penetrates the hair shaft, making it more porous and prone to extreme dryness. New growth starts to show within a few weeks.

Use an at-home conditioning treatment. And pin-curl or wrap your hair at night instead of rolling it.

Climate Control

Hot Weather

Summer hair should be carefree, in both styling and upkeep. Follow these pointers to minimize the effects of heat, humidity and the sun's damaging rays:

• Use moisturizing shampoos and conditioners to counteract the dehydration caused by the heat.

• Avoid overusing heating implements such as curling irons, flat irons and blow-dryers, which will cause dry, brittle hair.

• Maintain regular trims and touch-ups, and stick with lightweight styling products that will control frizz.

• Look for products with UV filters, vitamins and antioxidants to protect your hair from the sun. Ultraviolet rays from the sun can damage the protein structure of your hair.

• Wear a hat or scarf while sunning.

• Before taking a dip, slip on a swim cap and/or coat your hair with a leave-in conditioner to protect your hair from chlorine or salt.

• Rinse your hair with fresh water as soon as you emerge from the pool or ocean.

• Give your hair an intensive treatment once a week with a deep-cleansing shampoo and a nourishing mask.

Cold Weather

In cold-weather climates, winter's harsh winds, dry air and frigid temperatures can be brutal on tender strands. So you'll need to give your hair more moisture and attention to keep it healthy. Here's how to protect your hair from the big chill:

• Put your hair on winter bed rest. Roller-setting your coif is much less damaging than frequent blow-dryer styling.

• Schedule a deep-conditioning treatment when you're coloring, touching-up or getting a weave or braids. Deep conditioning helps your hair stay pliable, supple and shiny.

• Extend your touch-ups. This time of year the fewer chemical treatments your hair underg the better. Stretch that new-growth period from six to eight weeks to eight to ten weeks.

Distressed Tresses

Save Your Strands and Scalp

The condition of our hair reflects how we are taking care of ourselves—inside and out. Excessive shedding, flaking or breaking are indications that you need a checkup. If you see signs of distress, it's always a good idea to consult a dermatologist.

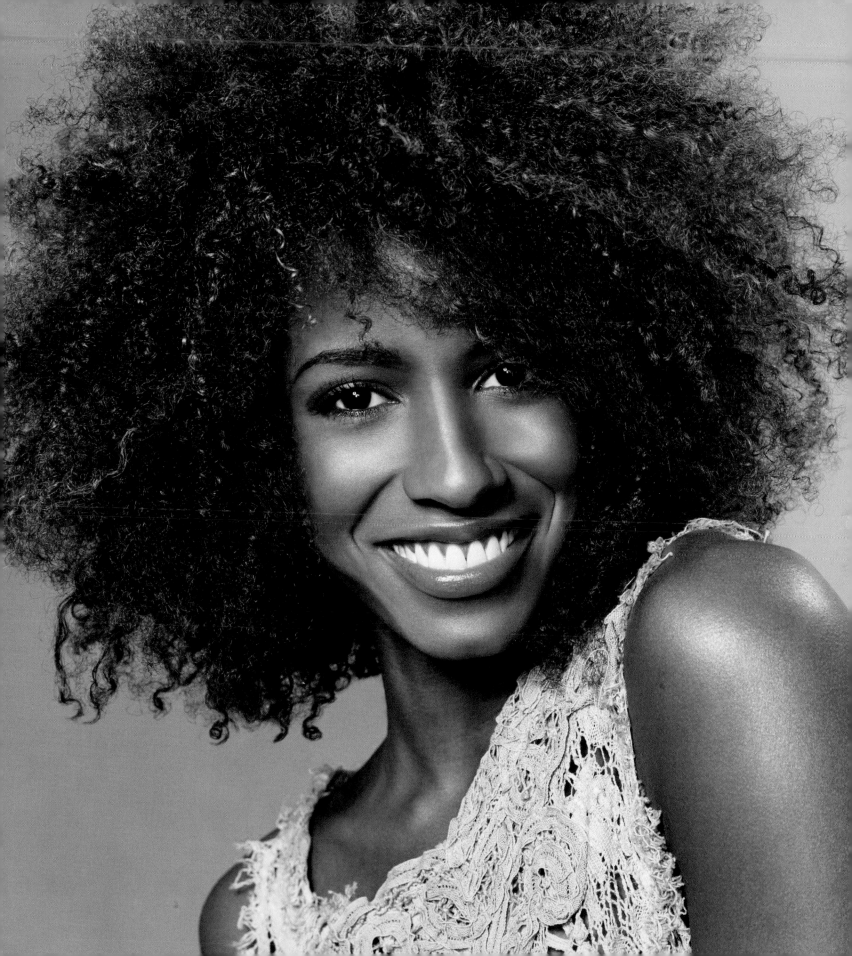

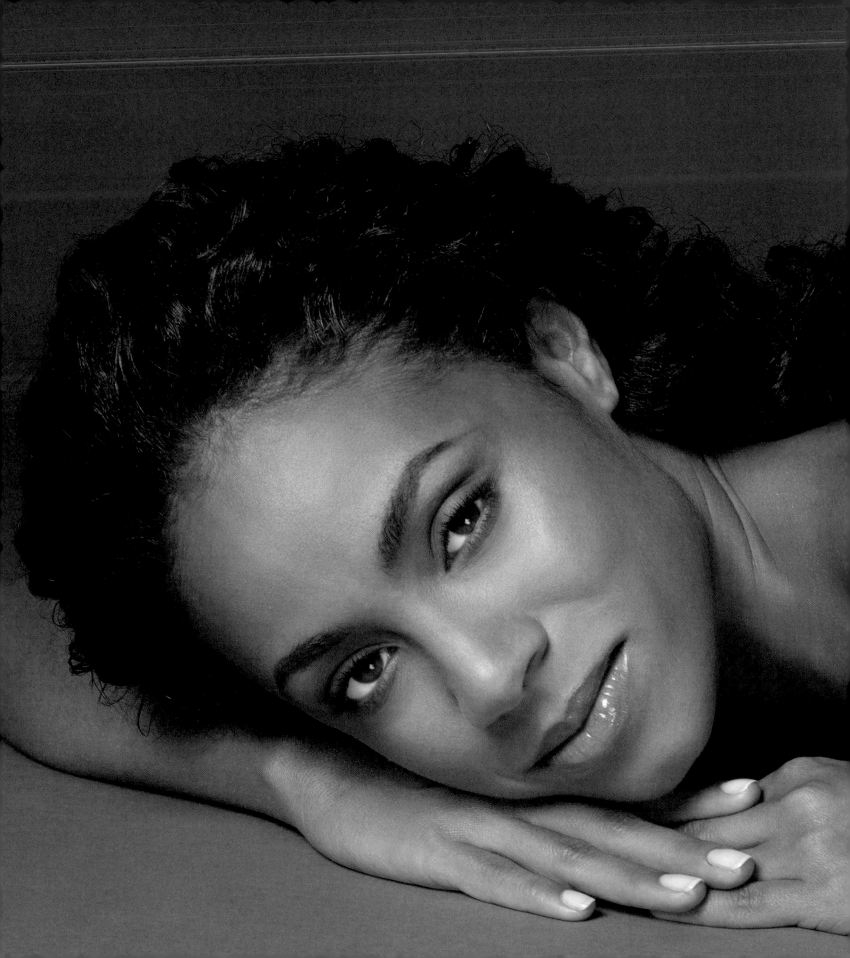

Healthy Skin

Throughout time writers have rhapsodized about the beauty of Black women's skin. With delicious descriptions they have told the world how gorgeous we are. From vanilla cream, caramel treat, café au lait and honey gold to brown sugar, cocoa and sepia, our beautiful hues inspire.

From face to feet, lusciously soft skin is our goal. But with our busy lives, we sometimes don't give our skin the time and attention needed to sustain its health and radiance. Our skin is as individual as we are, and critical to keeping it soft and supple is getting to know it well—how to nourish our skin and also recognize what irritates it. First, let's look at the big picture.

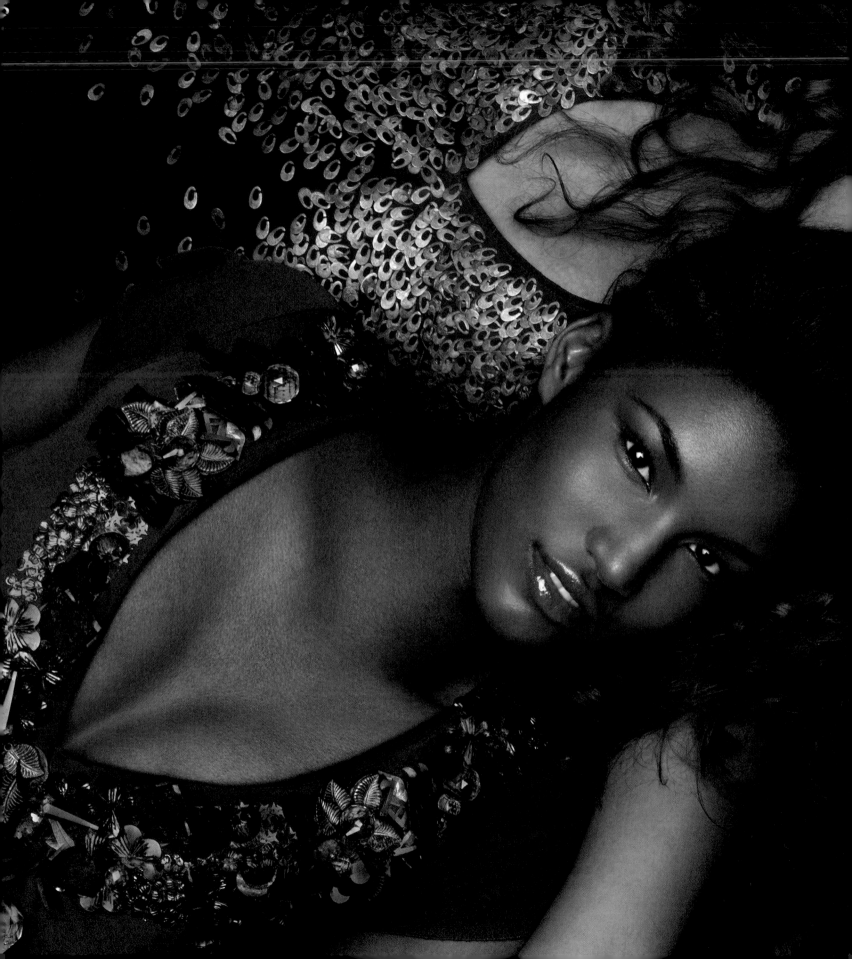

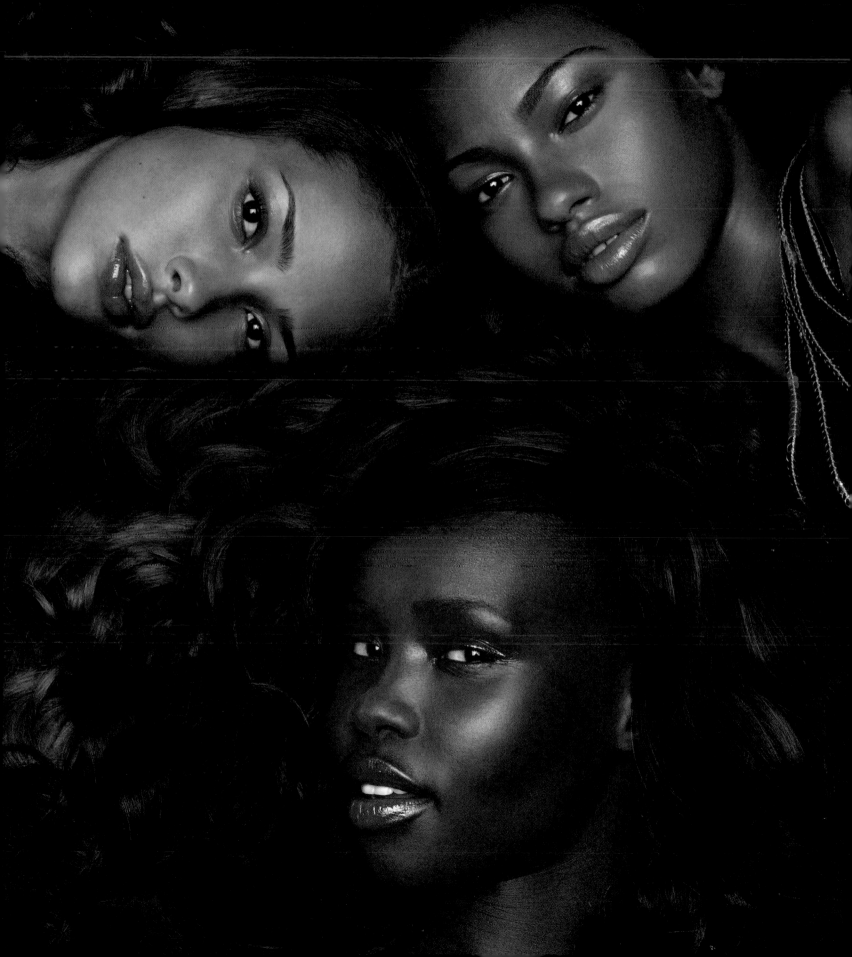

Basically Speaking

Your skin type can change based on internal factors such as your health, diet and stress level, or external things such as the season or climate where you live. Know the changes your skin may go through so that you can address them accordingly.

The skin is our body's major multitasker, defending us from environmental ravages, regulating body temperature, and insulating and cushioning our organs. Our skin works hard. Like the heart, lungs and liver, skin is an organ—our largest organ—and is composed of three distinct parts: the epidermis, dermis and subcutaneous layer.

The *epidermis,* the outer layer, is the one we are most preoccupied with since it is what's visible to the world. Here, skin cells are in a constant state of shedding and regeneration. Amazingly, we lose 30,000 to 40,000 dead cells from the surface of our skin each minute as newer cells move up to replace them. The epidermis also makes melanin, the substance that gives skin its color and protects it from the sun.

The *dermis,* the middle layer, is where nerve endings, blood vessels and oil and sweat glands are located. The dermis also contains collagen, the protein that is responsible for our skin's strength, and elastin, which is responsible for the skin's elasticity.

The *subcutaneous layer,* the underlying and deepest one, is primarily made up of fat to keep us warm and absorb shock.

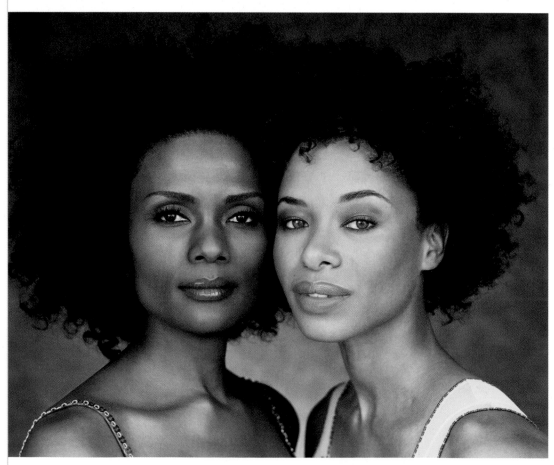

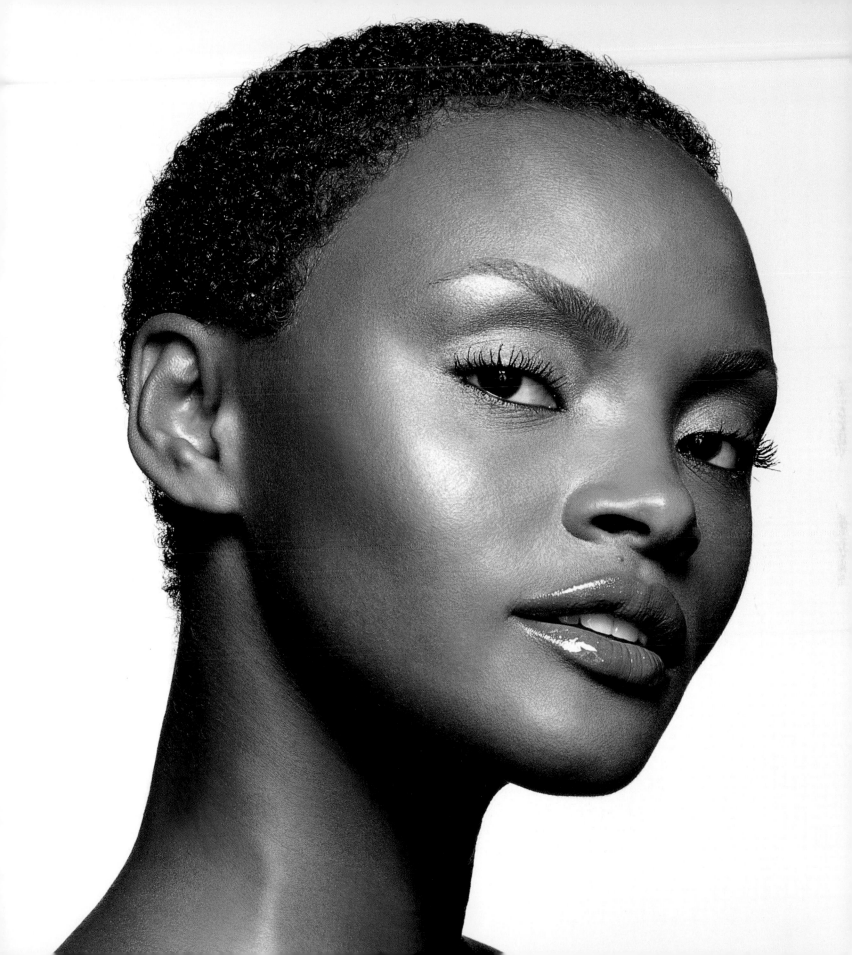

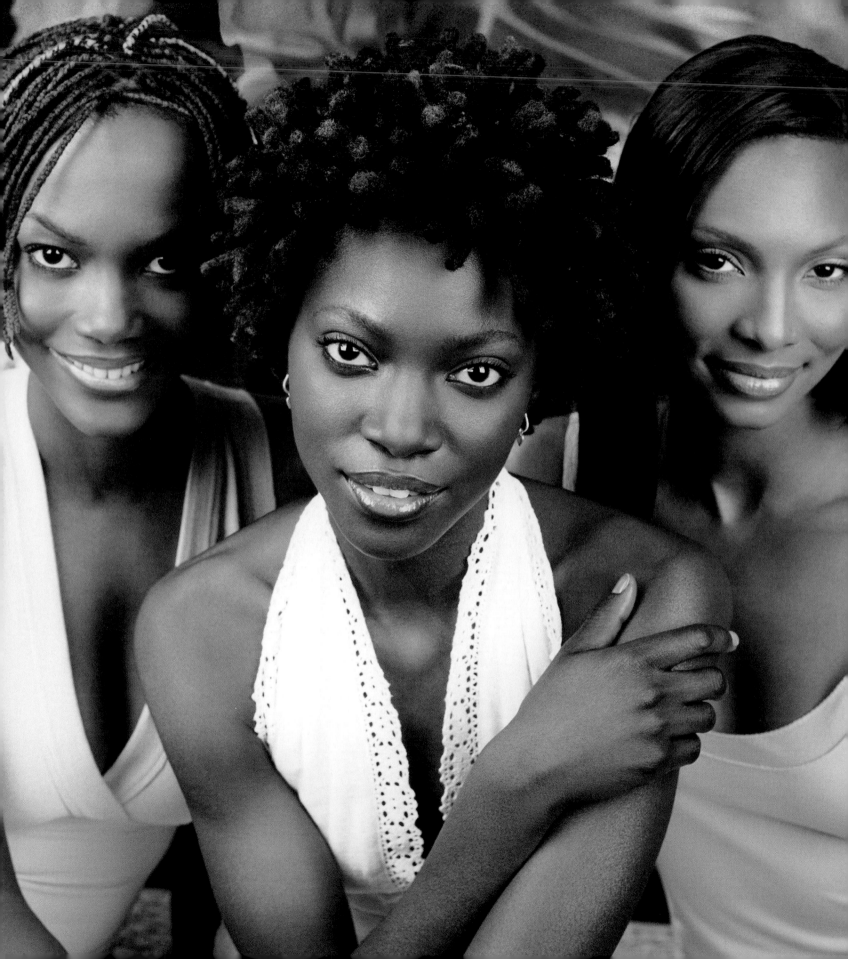

What's Your Type?

Our facial skin is a barometer of our general well-being. The products we use, the foods we eat and certainly our emotional state all affect our skin. Determine the type of skin you have, and incorporate the treatments that work best for you into your skin-care routine.

If Your Face Is Dry

Dry skin appears dull and ashen and tends to flake. It can feel tight and look dehydrated during winter and summer months, with fine lines becoming more noticeable.

- *Best cleanser:* A creamy formula that contains glycerin, hyaluronic acid or less than 10 percent lactic acid
- *Best moisturizer:* A superrich and creamy moisturizer
- *Best sunscreen:* An SPF formula of 15 to 30

If Your Face Is Oily

Oily skin is prone to breakouts, especially during the summer when the skin's natural oil production increases—because oil glands are more active in humid, warm weather. This skin type often has visible pores and surface shine.

- *Best cleanser:* A gel or foamy formula that contains salicylic acid or low concentrations of glycolic acid
- *Best moisturizer:* An oil-free brand made especially for oily skin that is unscented and free of lanolin and mineral oil
- *Best astringent:* Try toners first; if not effective try astringent
- *Best sunscreen:* An SPF formula of 15 to 30

If Your Face Is Combination Oily—Dry

Oily areas tend to occur along your face's T-zone—the nose, forehead and chin—with dry patches on the cheeks. An increase in the skin's natural oil production during the summer makes skin prone to breakouts during warmer months.

- *Best cleanser:* A cream or gel formula created for normal to dry skin
- *Best moisturizer:* An oil-free moisturizer on oilier areas and a dry-skin moisturizer on dry ones, or a combination-skin moisturizer
- *Best astringent:* An alcohol-based product only on oily areas
- *Best sunscreen:* An SPF formula of 30

If Your Face Is Sensitive

Sensitive skin is more easily affected by environmental factors and artificial ingredients in skin-care products. It's prone to irritation, sunburn, heat rashes and eczema.

- *Best cleanser:* A soap- and fragrance-free cleanser formulated for sensitive skin
- *Best moisturizer:* A hypoallergenic moisturizer for sensitive skin
- *Best sunscreen*: An SPF formula of 15 to 45, labeled for sensitive skin

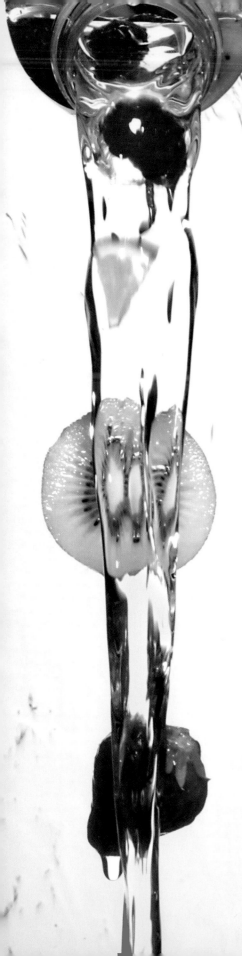

Skin-Enhancing Vitamins

Vitamin A: Vitamin A is an antioxidant that promotes new cell growth, aids in the repair of skin tissue and prevents some skin disorders, including acne.
• *Best Sources:* Green and yellow fruits and vegetables, liver and fish-liver oils

Vitamin B Complex
B1 (Thiamine): Thiamine is an antioxidant.
• *Best Sources:* Brown rice, egg yolks, fish, legumes, liver, peanuts, peas, poultry, pork, rice bran, wheat germ and whole grains

B2 (Riboflavin): This vitamin facilitates skin tissue's use of oxygen.
• *Best Sources:* Brown rice, egg yolks, fish, legumes, liver, peanuts, peas, poultry, pork, rice bran, wheat germ and whole grains

B3 (Niacin, Nicotinic Acid, Niacinamide): Niacin is important in maintaining healthy skin.
• *Best Sources:* Beef liver, brewer's yeast, broccoli, carrots, cheese, corn, flour, dandelion greens, wheat germ, dates, eggs, fish, tomatoes, pork, potatoes, peanuts and whole-wheat products

B5 (Pantothenic Acid): Concentrated in the body's organs, it is necessary for cellular health.
• *Best Sources:* Beef, brewer's yeast, eggs, fresh vegetables, kidney, legumes, liver, mushrooms, nuts, pork, royal jelly, saltwater fish, torula yeast, whole rye flour and whole wheat

B6 (Pyridoxine): It promotes red blood cell formation and normal cellular growth, and aids in the absorption of vitamin B12.
• *Best Sources:* Brewer's yeast, carrots, chicken, eggs, fish, meat, peas, spinach, sunflower seeds, walnuts and wheat germ

B12 (Cyanocobalamin): This vitamin is required for proper digestion and food absorption; it also aids in cellular growth and longevity.
• *Best Sources:* Brewer's yeast, clams, eggs, herring, kidney, liver, mackerel, dairy products and seafood

Biotin: Biotin maintains healthy skin and aids in cell growth.
• *Best Sources:* Brewer's yeast, cooked egg yolks, meat, milk, poultry, saltwater fish, soybeans and whole grains

Vitamin C: An antioxidant, vitamin C aids in tissue growth and repair; is essential in the formation of collagen; and promotes the healing of wounds, burns and bruises.
• *Best Sources:* Berries, citrus fruits and green vegetables

Vitamin E: Vitamin E is an antioxidant necessary for tissue repair; it also promotes healing, reduces scarring from some abrasions and promotes healthy skin.
• *Best Sources:* Cold pressed vegetable oils, dark leafy vegetables, legumes, nuts, seeds and whole grains

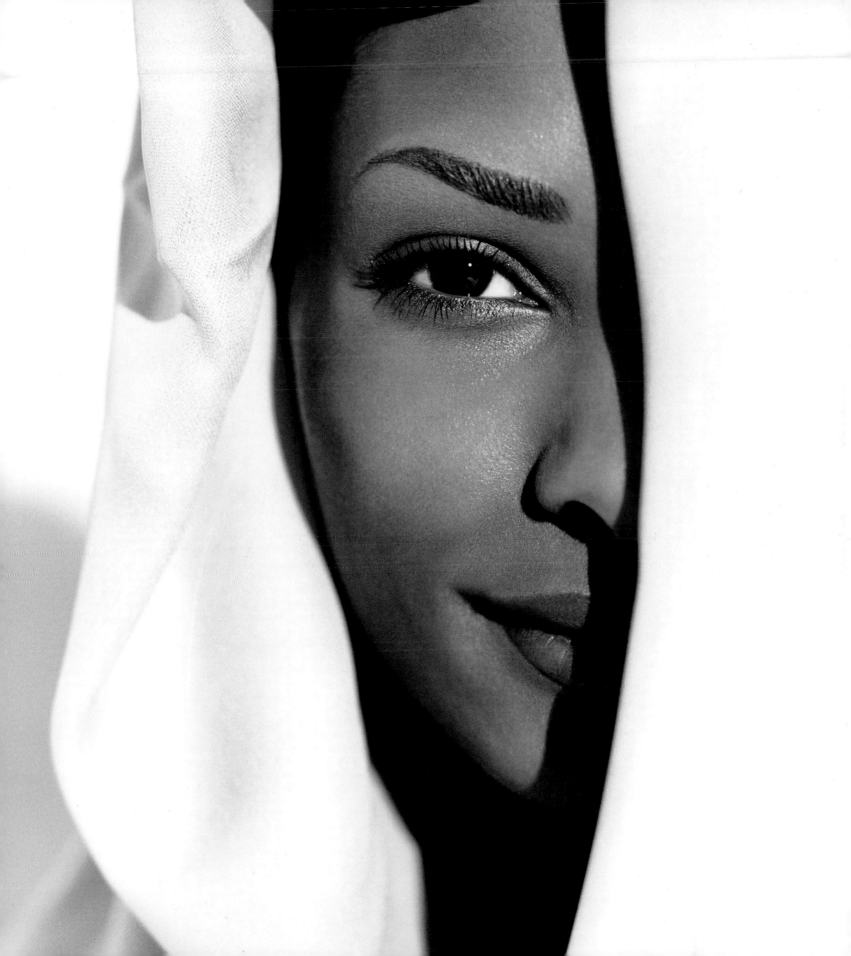

Wash with warm water to keep pores open and cleanse them; then rinse with cooler water to close your pores.

Never exfoliate using a formula containing crushed nuts, which can cut and damage skin.

Healthy Skin at Every Age

Today our skin has to work hard to stay healthy. Pollution, toxins, UV rays, cigarette smoke, stress—these are just some of the culprits that irritate our skin and cause fibrous tissue—elastin and collagen, which give skin its structure—to break down. Premature aging is the result. Technology is on our side, however. Today we have unlimited skin-care options. Here's the tried and true information to keep your skin healthy and clear.

Come Clean

It's important to cleanse your face twice daily, in the morning and before bedtime. Cleansers containing 1 to 2 percent salicylic or up to 10 percent glycolic acid work wonders on acne-prone skin. If dryness is a problem, look for ingredients like lactic acid, glycerin or hyaluronic acid. Sensitive skin types benefit from cleansers that are soap- and fragrance-free. Listen to your body. Discontinue using any product that irritates your skin. Apply your cleanser using an upward, circular motion, with a very soft washcloth or your hands. Use lukewarm water, taking care not to rub too hard or pull the delicate areas near your eyes. Rinse thoroughly, at least 20 times with cool water, and pat dry with a soft towel.

Exfoliate

Cleansing, toning and moisturizing your skin aren't enough—you have to go deeper, especially if you have oily skin. Sometimes the old dry and dull skin hangs on, dulling your complexion and clogging pores. Oily skin is a magnet for dead skin. And as we age, the skin's renewal

6 Skin Savers

➤ **Invest in two moisturizers** to care for your skin properly. Good ones will protect it and keep it from getting dry, sallow and lackluster. You need a daily moisturizer with an SPF of at least 15 to 30—no matter what your complexion. Besides safeguarding against skin cancer, sunscreen can prevent melasma (mask of pregnancy) and hyperpigmentation. At night, use an SPF-free moisturizer that intensively treats your top skin concern (acne, aging, dry or oily skin).

➤ **Avoid sleeping on your face.** This position encourages irritation from hair-product residue on your pillowcase.

➤ **Treat your skin to monthly facials.** A professional cleansing is the best way to keep skin clear and breakouts at bay. A good aesthetician will address any antiaging concerns and advise you on the latest treatments for specific skin conditions, such as uneven texture and tone and adult acne.

➤ **Don't smoke.** Besides releasing some thousand-odd toxins onto your skin, smoking constricts blood vessels and deprives skin of the oxygen it needs to stay radiant and healthy.

➤ **Don't yo-yo diet.** Gaining and losing weight puts stress on skin's elasticity, and, over time, the skin won't spring back into shape as readily.

➤ **Invest in a gentle scrub.** Look for one with superfine granules and/or enzymes to buff away and dissolve dead cells and leave your skin renewed and aglow.

mechanism slows down. Exfoliating speeds up the renewal process, sloughing away dead skin and revealing the plumper, more radiant new cells. When sloughing becomes part of your beauty ritual, your skin gets smoother and more evenly toned. You can exfoliate manually with scrubs and grains. Or you can use over-the-counter preparations that contain enzymes, acids and chemicals that exfoliate. If you have oily skin, you may want to exfoliate every other night. The driest skin should be exfoliated weekly.

If you are plagued by uneven skin tone and texture, you may want to consider professionally administered microdermabrasion or chemical peels. Microdermabrasion uses aluminum oxide or sodium bicarbonate crystals to remove dead skin, while chemical peels use compounds like fruit acids to speed up the shedding process. Treatments typically cost $100 to $250. Exfoliators once reserved for professional use only are now available at drugstores and cosmetics counters. These products are usually safe for at-home use and are often just a step up from basic scrubs. For best results, however, we recommend going to a professional, an aesthetician or dermatologist, who is experienced in working with Black skin.

Tone Up

You can use an astringent or toner or freshener after washing your face to remove any trace of makeup or pollution. Toners and fresheners recommended for dry to normal skin usually are mild and contain no alcohol. Astringents best for oily skin normally contain alcohol, which is more drying to the skin. Both can work to restore skin's pH balance.

Experts are split on whether these products are necessary. The high-caliber cleansers on the market today do an excellent job of removing makeup and debris, and skin will naturally return to its proper pH balance. If your skin is excessively oily and prone to breakouts, you may benefit from an astringent, especially during the summer months when your skin's oil glands are most active. If you have combination skin, and you think this type of product would be helpful, use a toner only on the oily areas. If you experience any burning, stinging

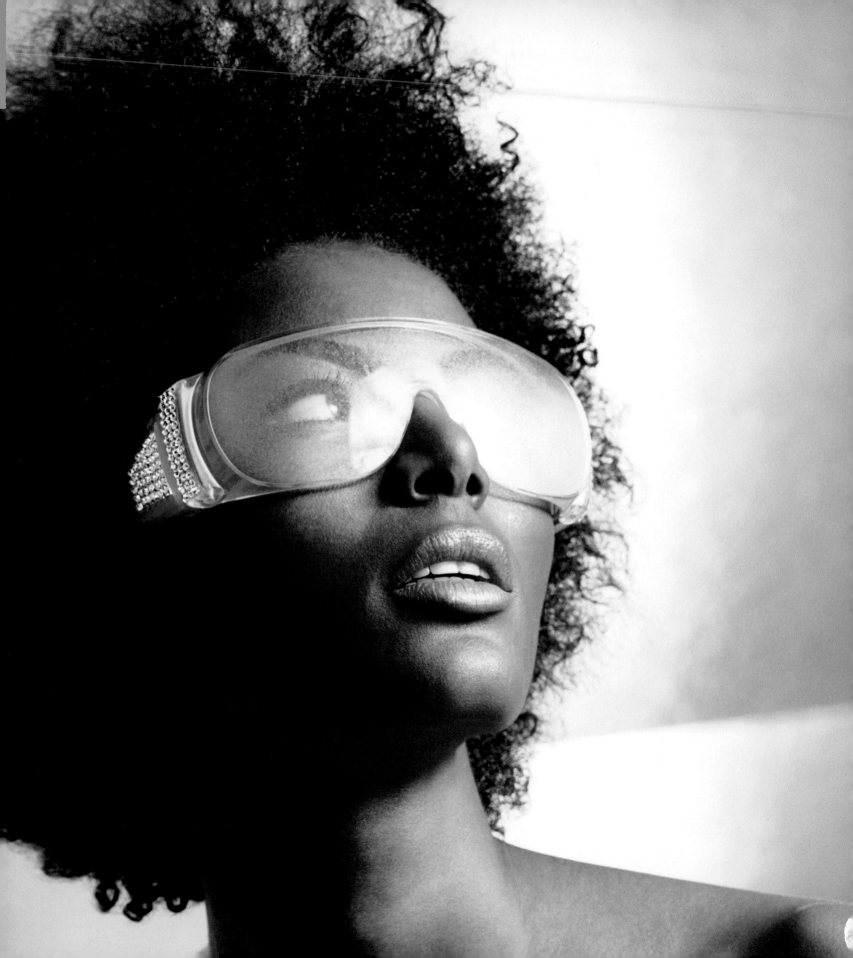

or irritation, switch back to a milder formulation made specifically for sensitive skin, or skip astringents and toners altogether.

Moisturize

All skin types need regular moisturizing with humectants, ingredients that attract water from the atmosphere to the skin. Generally, creams contain the highest percentage of humectants, followed by lotions, then balms and gels. Choose based on your skin's needs for moisture. Creams and lotions are best for dry skin. Balms and gels are recommended for oily and combination skin. Know your skin type, and read labels so that you select formulations designed specifically for you.

Traditionally, skin-care experts have recommended moisturizing your skin twice daily after cleansing. Now some say applying moisturizer before bedtime is not necessary, that your skin needs a chance to breathe. Listen to your skin. If it's dry and flaky in the morning, you need to smooth on a rich moisturizer before going to bed.

One rule never to bend: Always use a moisturizer with an SPF of 15 to 30 for dark to medium skin tones and above 30 for lighter skin before applying foundation—even on a cloudy day.

Protect

For years, we Black folks ignored how crucial it is to safeguard our skin from the sun's ultraviolet rays, opting instead to believe that our melanin would protect us. And it does, but only to a certain extent. Yes, Black can crack. Even the darkest-skinned people who work or bathe in the sun for years will be wrinkled in old age. The extremely harmful results of prolonged sun exposure might appear decades after we boldly basked in the sun. According to studies, Black women diagnosed with nonmelanoma skin cancer are seven and a half times more likely than White women with the same disease to develop an additional form of cancer. And though fewer of us will ever suffer from skin cancer, we are not immune to it. So no matter how fabulously dark you are, before stepping out—whether to the office or the beach—play it safe by smoothing on sunscreen over all your exposed areas.

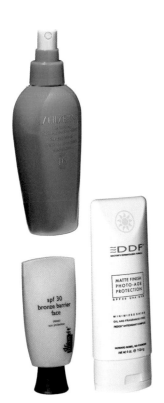

Sunscreen Tips

➤ Look for broad- or full-spectrum sunblocks. These protect against both ultraviolet alpha (UVA) rays, which cause premature aging and skin cancer, and ultraviolet beta (UVB) rays, which are mainly responsible for sunburns that can also result in skin cancer. Our melanin provides some added protection against UVB rays, but it gives no additional safeguard against UVA rays.

➤ Use sunblocks with an SPF of 15 to 30 for everyday wear. If you plan to be outside for more than a few hours, an SPF of 30 or higher is best.

➤ Proper application is key. Apply sunblock 20 minutes before going outside, and reapply it every two hours.

➤ Remember to apply more sunblock to sensitive areas—around your eyes, nose and ears.

➤ Refresh your sunblock supply annually. Most have a shelf life of one year.

A Guide to Power- house Ingredients

Today's antiaging creams promise firmer, younger, smoother skin. Many are just hype. But scientific breakthroughs have led to products that work to protect and repair the skin. Here are some of the latest and greatest ingredients to know.

Alpha Hydroxy Acids

Also referred to as AHAs, alpha hydroxy acids are effective chemical exfoliators that help smooth, clarify and even skin tone. Two of the most commonly used AHAs, glycolic and lactic acids, detach dry skin cells and allow the healthy shedding of dead skin. However, these can be irritating, especially in concentrations higher than 10 percent.

Antioxidants

Vitamins A, C and E, grapeseed extract, green tea, white tea, pomegranate, soy and coenzyme Q10 are a few of the varieties of antioxidants now available. They inhibit the damage caused by free radicals (skin-destroying elements caused by sun, smoke and other environmental pollutants).

Hyaluronic Acid

This element also occurs naturally in skin. It contains water-binding properties that provide moisture to skin.

Peptides

These are strings of amino acids that renew the skin's outer layer by accelerating the development of newer cells. Peptides have also been clinically proven to stimulate the production of collagen and elastin and reduce the appearance of wrinkles.

Retinoids

Derivatives of vitamin A, retinoids stimulate cell turnover and reduce clumping, resulting in refined skin texture and a more even tone.

Soy Extracts

Some products use soy extracts for their lightening benefits. Although these agents are not as powerful as synthetic chemicals such as hydroquinone and kojic acid, their bleaching effects occur over an extended period of time.

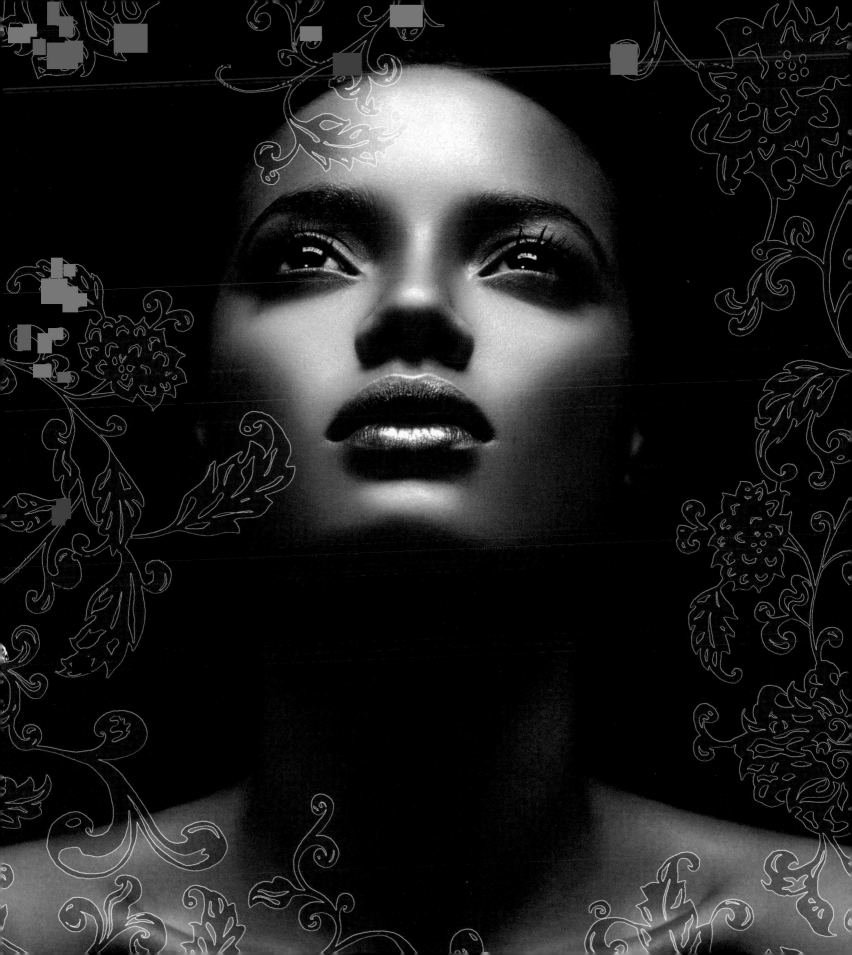

9 Bad Habits
That Stand Between You and Great Skin

1 Touching your face throughout the day—this habit is one of the major sources of breakouts and rashes.

2 Wearing oil-based makeup and moisturizers—these formulas tend to clog your pores.

3 Sleeping with makeup—make sure your skin is super-clean overnight so that it benefits from your body's natural restorative work while you sleep.

4 Using greasy pomades and oily hair sprays—these can run onto the face and cause breakouts.

5 Drinking too little water—dehydrated skin is dull, so drink 8 to 10 eight-ounce glasses of water a day to hydrate skin and flush out impurities.

6 Skipping the sunblock—wear it anytime you're outdoors, even on cloudy days.

7 Stressing out—stress causes worry and frown lines, and it produces hormones that wreak havoc on your skin.

8 Not eating several servings of fruits and vegetables each day—they are the best natural source of vitamins and antioxidants, which protect skin cells by neutralizing damaging and aging free radicals.

9 Diagnosing and treating breakouts and rashes yourself—see a dermatologist at the onset of any irritation to prevent further eruptions.

Professional Care

Skin is a miracle. It's in a constant state of renewal, shedding dead skin cells about every 28 days. But pollution, stress, sun exposure and some foods can have an adverse effect on our complexion. Having regular deep-cleansing facials help remove dead-cell buildup, rejuvenate the skin and keep it functioning properly.

Depending on the state of your skin and your skin type, a facial should include steaming; black- and whitehead extraction; a rejuvenating, moisturizing or oil-reducing mask; and a massage. Today, some facialists are incorporating extras like oxygen therapy and acupressure. After a facial, your skin should feel glorious, look clean and hydrated, and be glowing.

Ask family, friends and coworkers for the best aesthetician in town who works with lots of Black clients. If this approach doesn't turn up an expert, do your own due diligence, keeping these tips in mind:

Make sure the facialist is licensed. A quality aesthetician should be state certified (meaning that she has at least 300 hours of training). Postgraduate study and a working knowledge of the latest industry advances are big pluses. Over the phone, ask about any specialties. And don't equate the number of years in the business with quality service. Consistently upgrading skills and expertise in treating our skin are key.

Schedule a consultation. Check on the environment to make sure it's clean and pleasant. Let the aesthetician look at your skin without makeup, evaluate it and make a recommendation. Be sure that your concerns are listened to and the results you want are understood.

Ask questions. An expert should be able to easily answer questions about the specific treatments provided, as well as about the tools used and at-home skin care.

Make sure you feel at ease. Trust your instincts. If you feel good about the aesthetician's expertise and comfortable in your exchanges, make an appointment for the end of the day or on the weekend, and try skipping makeup for a day or two after your facial.

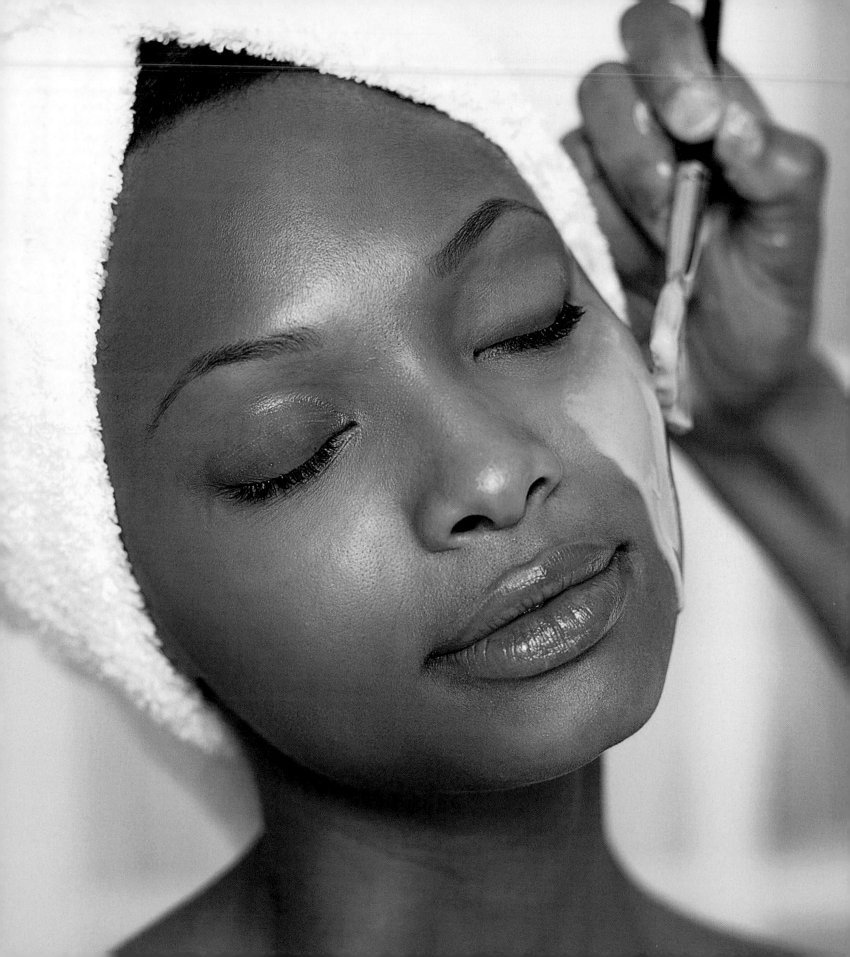

Everything about Facials & Masks

Choosing the Best Facial for Your Skin

One of the best perks of getting a facial is the fact that it's customized to address your skin's specific needs. Whether your issue is breakouts, lackluster skin, dark spots or simply maintenance of already good skin, there are treatments for everyone. But remember: Since your skin does change, the products and methods used should also change when necessary. Here are some general treatment guidelines to know before you go.

Enzyme Peels

For: Acne-prone or sensitive skin

Results: Pore-clogging bacteria and sebum are released with little irritation.

Facial for Dry Skin

For: Sagging skin

Results: Oxygen facials deliver oxygen to the cells to fight damaging free radicals, which break down the skin's structure and elasticity, so skin appears firmer. Collagen facials improve subtleness and lessen the appearance of fine lines.

Alpha and Beta Hydroxy Acids

For: Aging skin

Results: Treatments with these ingredients help skin cells regenerate faster, by exfoliating dull, dry dead cells and revealing plumper and radiant new ones beneath them.

3 Tips for Getting a Facial

To prevent having a bad facial experience, it's important to do your homework and investigate your options. Here are some facts to keep in mind:

➤ Don't let an aesthetician do the work of a dermatologist. Only a dermatologist should perform procedures like laser treatments, certain techniques that remove entire layers of skin, Botox injections and pimple lancing.

➤ Tell your aesthetician immediately if a treatment starts to burn, itch or irritate your skin. Let her know whether she is applying too much pressure during an extraction. Harsh handling of the skin can cause scarring, discoloration, broken capillaries and other damage.

➤ Share important details. Be sure to let the aesthetician know whether you are using medications like Retin-A or glycolics that could interfere with a treatment.

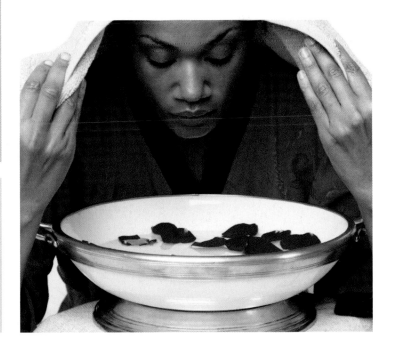

At-Home Facials

You won't be able to reproduce every step of an in-salon facial, and you should never try to extract pimples, but you can easily steam, cleanse, nourish and refresh your skin at home. Lots of products, both high-end and lower priced, offer great results. Also, you can always use natural ingredients from your kitchen. Try these recipes for a steaming sensation and masks for different skin types.

STEAM TREAT

1 gallon of distilled water

2 tablespoons of salt

¾ cup of peppermint leaves, or seven drops of peppermint essential oil

A large bowl

A towel

Facial mask (optional)

Toner or witch hazel (optional)

1. Boil water, adding two tablespoons of salt per gallon. Pour the boiling water over the peppermint leaves or oil in a temperature-safe bowl. Place your face 12 inches above the water, and use a towel to cover your head like a tent to keep the steam in. Alternate two minutes of steaming over the bowl with a two-minute break.

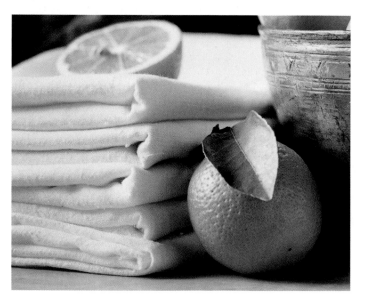

2. Repeat this cycle up to five times for a total of 10 minutes over steam. Rinse your face in lukewarm water. This is a good time to use a mud or peel-off facial mask made specifically for your skin type to get the maximum benefit while your pores are open.

3. Rinse your face again. Follow with a toner if you have dry skin or witch hazel if your skin is oily.

Make Your Mask

For Dry Skin:

AVOCADO MASK

Mash the pulp of a ripe avocado and apply it all over your face and throat. Allow it to sit for 10 minutes; then rinse with lukewarm water. Avocado is chock-full of proteins and amino acids. Your skin will feel smooth as silk.

PROTEIN MASK

Beat one egg white, and apply it to your face and throat. Leave on for 15 minutes and then rinse. Egg whites are a nourishing treat for dry and sensitive skin.

Oily and Combination Skin:

BANANA MASK

Mash a ripe banana in a bowl; add a tablespoon of honey and a few drops of orange or lemon juice. Mix ingredients to form a paste. Apply and leave on face for 15 minutes; then rinse with warm water. Banana calms your skin while the acids from the orange or lemon juice remove dry, flaky skin.

ACNE MASK

Blend equal amounts of fresh mint and cilantro in a food processor; add enough water to make a paste. Powdered zinc, available in health-food stores, will increase the anti-inflammatory benefits of the mixture.

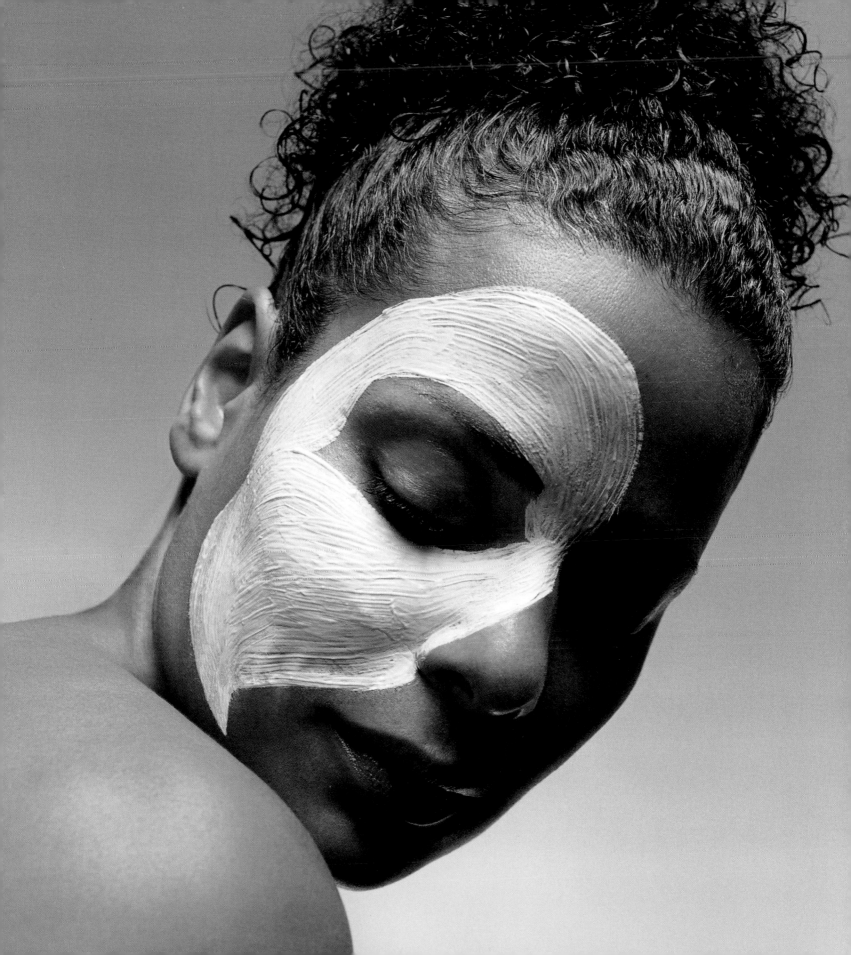

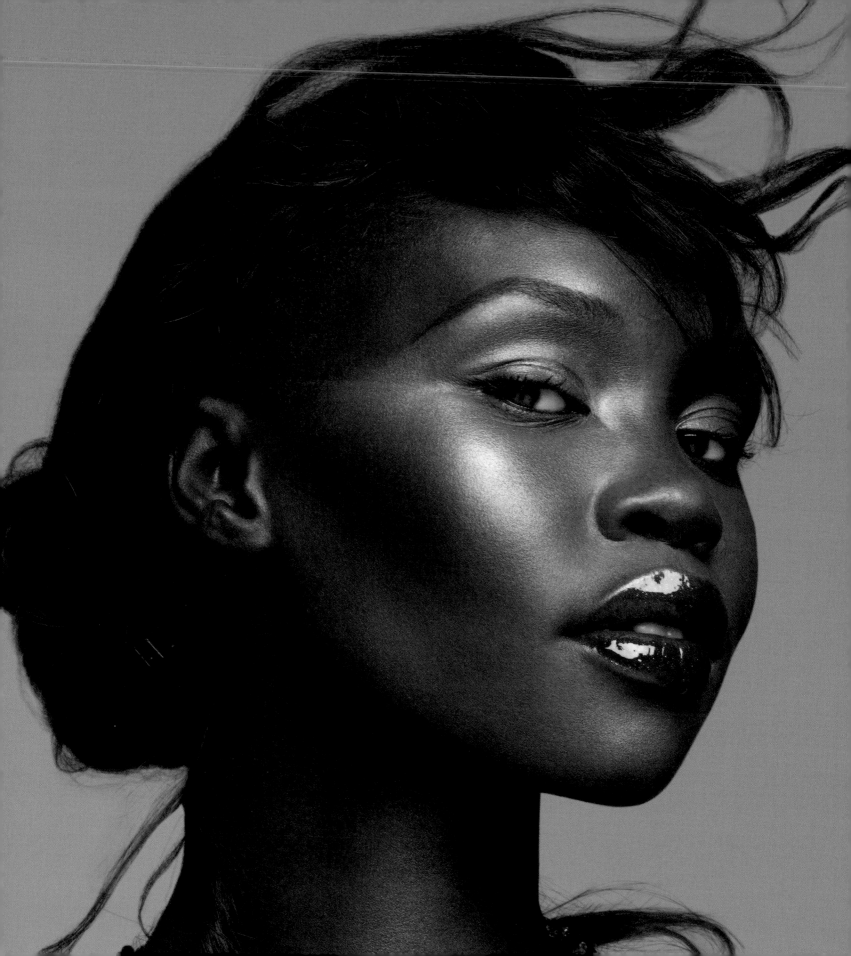

Making Faces

Today's makeup companies are spinning out more products with colors and textures made for us than ever before. From foundation shades to shadows that won't fade on you, the major cosmetic brands are marketing Black beauty, making it easier than ever for you to get your glam on. All you need are the right tools and tips. Read on for everything you'll want to know about makeup—from foundation to lip gloss.

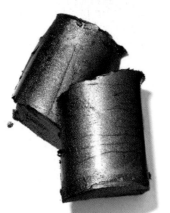

Foundation:
Choosing the Right One

Putting your best face forward really begins with healthy skin. The right foundation only makes good-looking skin look even better. And there's a banquet of foundation shades and textures for you to choose from. The newest ones come in natural-looking colors and formulas that ensure the perfect match, whether you want a little coverage or a lot. For a light finish, sheer liquids and tinted moisturizers do the trick, and for greater coverage, pressed powders and cream or stick foundations are perfect choices. Avoid the masklike "base face" of the seventies and eighties and apply foundation only where you need it—you don't want to cover up your glow. Looking natural is always the goal, and some of the newest formulations include light-reflecting pigments that mimic skin perfectly.

Tinted Moisturizers
If you want just a bit more of a dewy radiance and your natural skin to show through, try a tinted moisturizer. This light, barely-there formulation is blended with just a hint of color and is a great choice for a clean, fresh no-makeup look. Choose one with an SPF of 15 or higher to protect your skin from the sun's skin-damaging rays. One caveat: Most tinted moisturizers work best on ivory to warm golden-brown skin tones. The high titanium-dioxide content in many of these formulations causes an ashy appearance on deeper hues.

Liquid Foundation
Liquids are the largest category and offer Black women the most choices. Just peruse the cosmetics section of any department store or superdrugstore. Whether you have oily, dry or combination skin, want a little or a lot of coverage, have sensitive skin or want extra protection from the sun, you can find or create a formulation right for you.

Cream Foundation
Cream foundations offer super coverage, and you have to be a blend master when using them; otherwise they look heavy and masklike. Apply with a sponge and blend, blend, blend, thinning the cream and working it into your skin until it looks natural.

Stick Foundation
Stick foundations are excellent in covering hyperpigmentation, scars or any discoloration. Those with a suedelike texture—smooth and creamy—are easily blendable. In addition, a stick foundation can do double duty as a concealer and work well for spot coverage by itself or as a primer before applying other formulations or powder. Available in water-based and oil-free formulas, sticks offer medium to full coverage and usually a semi-matte finish.

Cream–Powder
A dream to use, cream-to-powder makeup glides on like a cream and dries to a powder finish. Great for all skin types, it offers a powdery matte finish and moderate coverage.

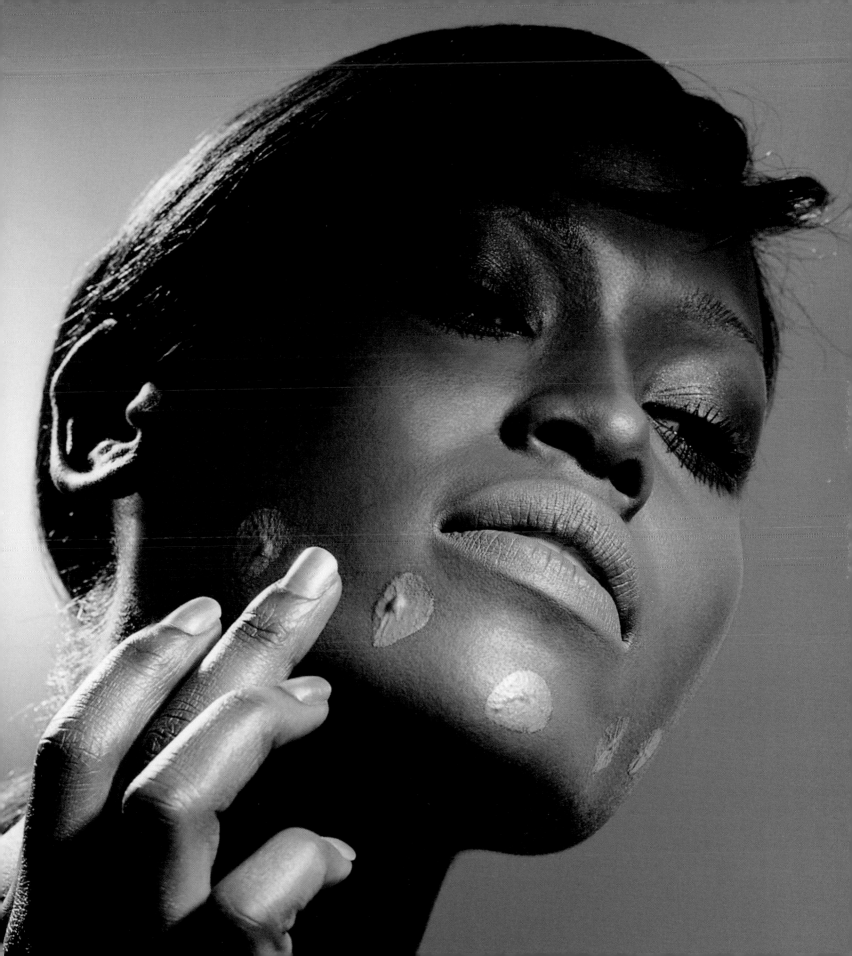

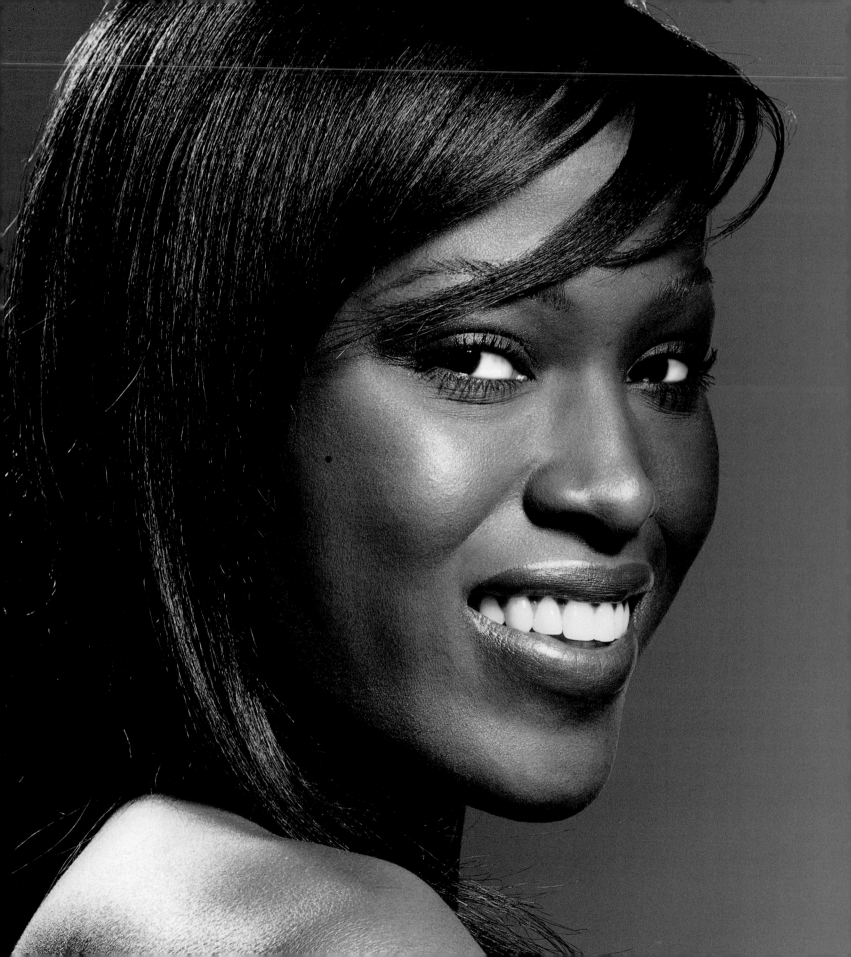

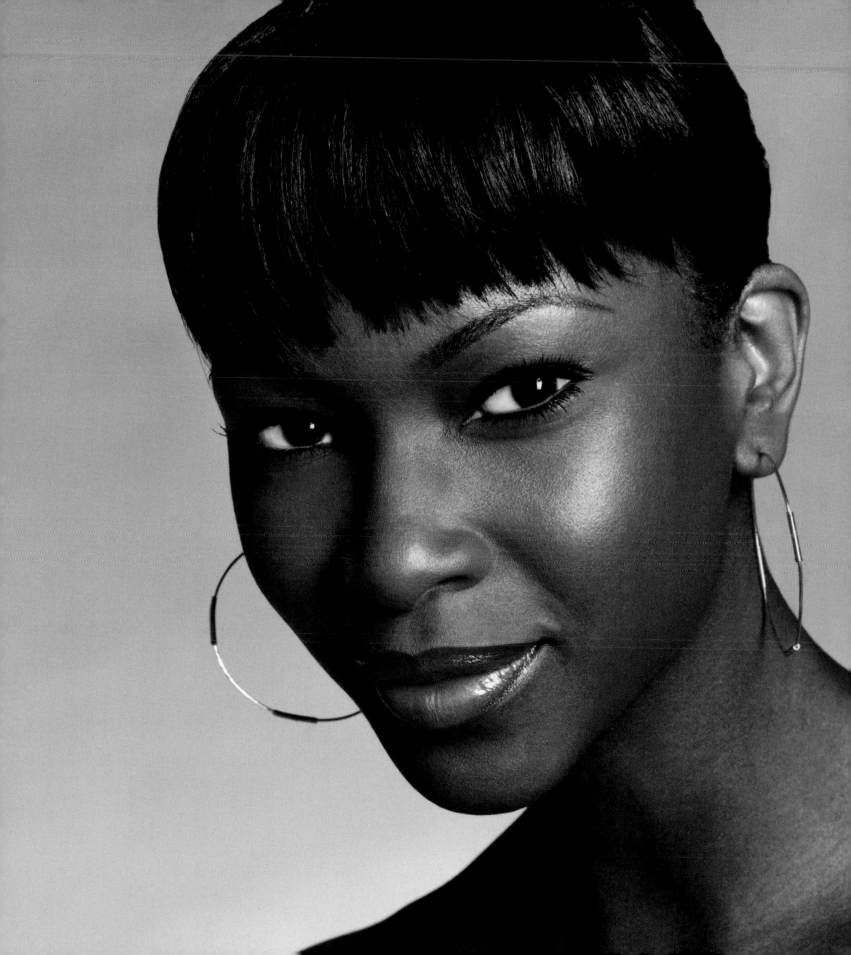

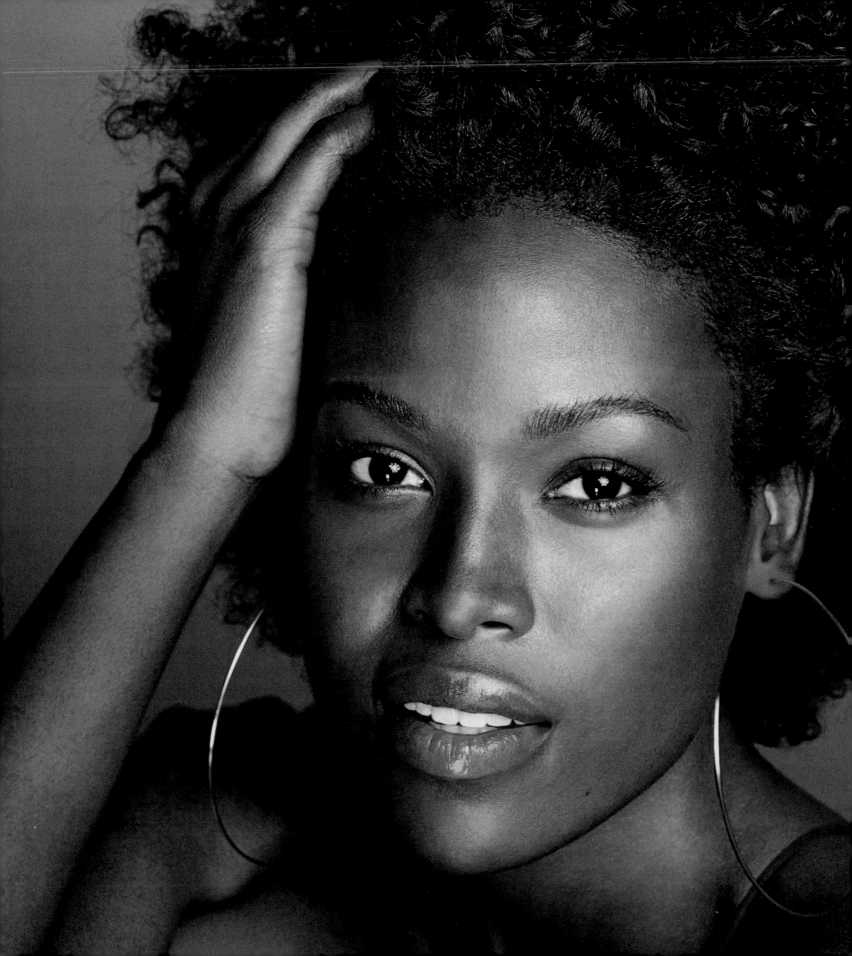

Ace Your Base

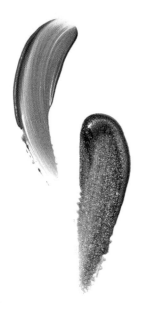

Follow these five foolproof tips to help you uncover your perfect match:

Determine your undertone. Your undertone is your skin's "underlying" color. It's easy to figure out and critical to know in order to choose natural-looking foundation. Here's what to do: Look at the inside of your wrist in natural light and you'll actually see a yellowish, reddish, greenish or bluish hue. Whichever color it is, is your undertone.

Identify the right hue for you. Perform a swatch test with the shade closest to your undertone and skin color. To ensure the perfect match, apply on one side of your face, step outside the store with a little mirror and view your selection in natural light. Walk around for a while and examine the color on your face again before purchasing it. Check to see if it's changed shades, which sometimes happens when pigments in foundation mix with the skin's natural oils. If you don't find a perfect match, buy a second shade, either lighter or darker, whatever you need. At home you can easily add a bit of the second shade to the primary one if you're working with liquid foundations. With creams and sticks you'll have to add a bit of the second shade to the basic one

in the palm of your hand or directly on your skin and blend them to perfection. This approach may seem complicated, but it's really not, and in a few days you'll master it.

Solve your skin concerns. If you have oily or acne-prone skin, look for foundations with oil-absorbing ingredients like silicone, salicylic acid and clay. Want to cover up scars, hyperpigmentation or birthmarks? Reach for a corrective cover-up or an opaque foundation. Need a long-lasting makeup that can hang with your 24–7 schedule? Consider a primer–foundation duo. The primer smoothes the skin's surface and controls the oil so that foundation glides on and adheres for enduring flawless complexion.

Know where to look. Not every cosmetic company has a range of shades extensive enough to match all of our many skin tones. If you have difficulty finding the perfect match, simply ask sisters your color whose makeup looks great what brands they shop.

Need more help? Shop where Black women or men are working at the cosmetic counters. They have the most expertise in understanding our needs.

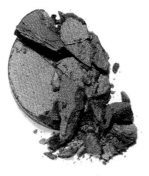

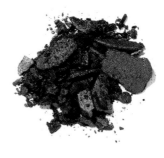

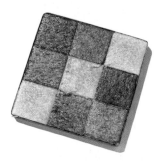

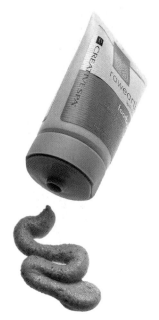

Powder: The Finishing Touch

Icing on the cake! Powder sets makeup, keeps it looking fresh and helps prevent shine. But use it sparingly; otherwise skin looks dry and unnatural. Look for powders that offer skin-care benefits. The newest type will self-adjust to oil and moisture or hydrate the skin with water-based technology.

Pressed Powder Compact and concentrated, pressed powder can be used solo to even and smooth skin and to matte shine. Used over foundation, it adds a smooth finish. Pressed powders tend to offer more opacity than loose ones, so use a very light touch. You may want to use just on oily areas or any part of your face you want to keep matte. What we love about pressed powder is that it comes in compact form, making touch-ups quick and easy anywhere.

Loose Powder Lighter in texture than pressed powder, loose powder leaves a more natural finish but is a bit messy to work with. Apply with a large brush. Shake excess powder (off the brush), and "dust" your skin using the lightest possible strokes.

Concealer: Hide and Sleek

Concealer is the big sister of the base family. Similar to foundation but heavier and more concentrated, concealers can cover and diminish imperfections. For example, they disguise dark undereye circles, pimples and dark marks. They are designed for use on specific areas, not all over the face, and are available in four forms of packaging.

Tube Creamy in texture, these offer medium coverage.

Pot Also creamy in texture but usually more opaque, they are best for dark marks and undereye circles.

Stick Stick concealers often look like lipstick and can be applied directly to a spot and blended for maximum to sheer coverage. They are not recommended for the eye area because they can drag on fragile skin.

Wand This type gives semisheer coverage. You can put the product directly on your skin with the applicator, then blend with a sponge.

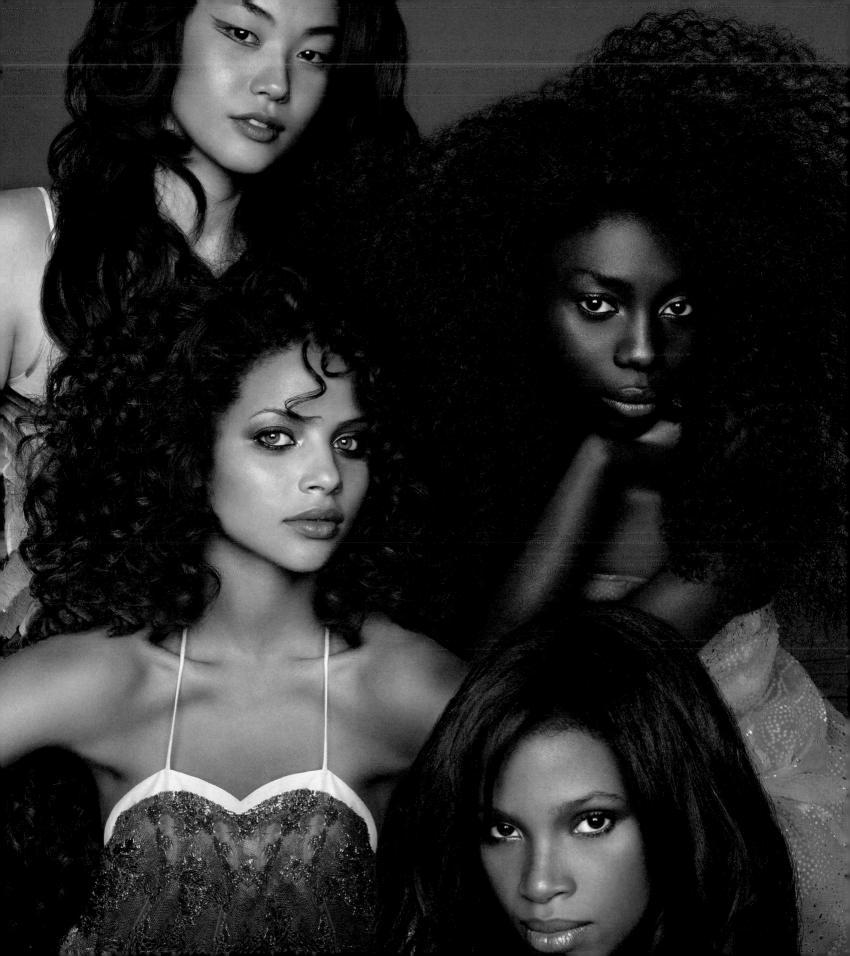

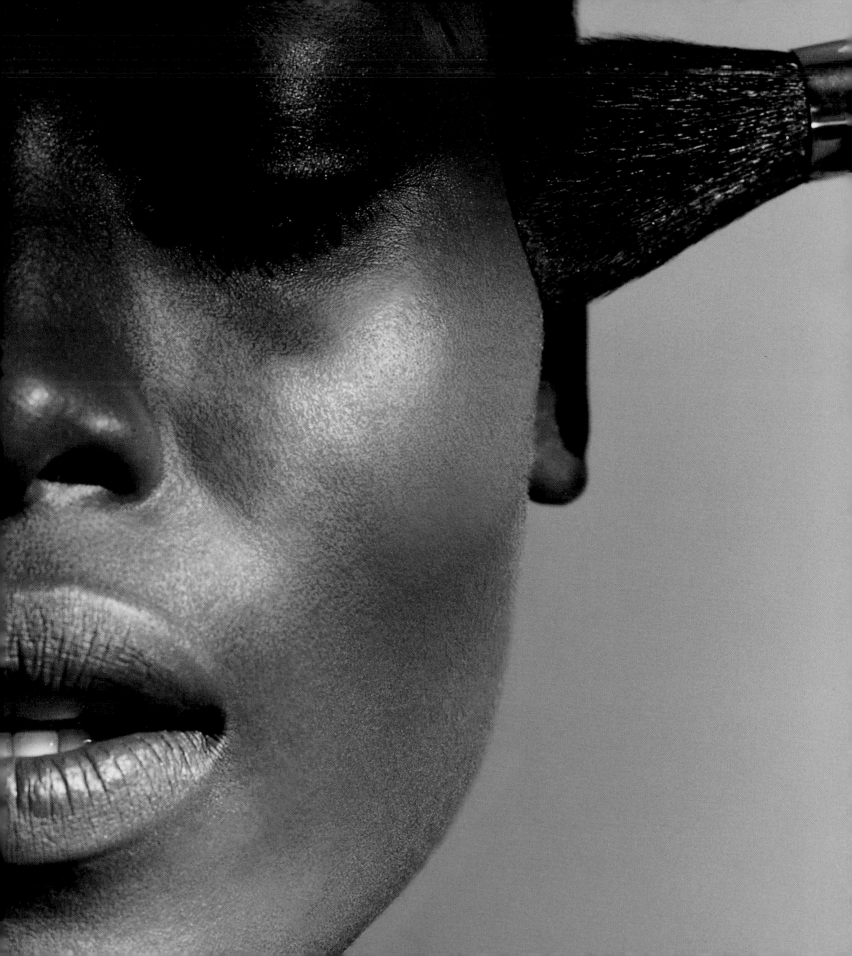

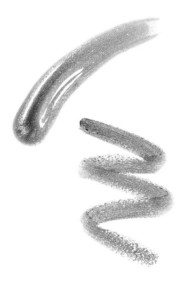

Remember that blush should look whisper-soft. Less is always more.

Blush: A Hint of Color

Blush is magic! It makes foundation look more natural, and even without foundation, blush can add a healthy glow to any complexion. Shades range from petal pink for the lightest skin tones to rich plum for the deepest ones, and they are available in textures as varied as sticks, gels and powders.

Blushing Beauty

Use this chart to help select just the right-colored blush to bring out your beautiful best.

Skin Color	Blush Color	Tip
Very light	Soft pinks	Browned pinks offer a rosy glow to fairer skin.
Medium light	Peach	Peach is a great neutral, especially lending a sunny cast to yellowish undertones.
Light-brown	Bronze	Warm bronzes are beautiful on golden skin tones.
Medium-brown	Orange and rosy	Caramel complexions look wonderful with warm oranges and muted roses.
Dark-brown	Plums and reds	Darker complexions look gorgeous with deep rich hues.
Deep-brown	Blue-reds	Rich bluish reds give deep-brown skin even more vibrancy.
Black-brown	Deep-burgundy and copper	Burgundy and copper can add a burst of natural color to beautiful Black skin.

Cheer Up Your Cheeks!

Choose a favorite formulation of blush that gives your skin a healthy glow.

Sticks render a more natural look than powder, are easy to use and give skin a dewy finish. Although the portable packaging is convenient, stick concealers dry faster than gels or creams, making them harder to blend. They are not the best for oily skin: Dewy plus oily can equal greasy. *Application:* For a seamless finish, dab just a bit on your cheeks and blend with a foundation brush.

Gels are transparent and lightweight, giving cheeks the sheerest hint of color. Because gel blushes are water-based and tend to evaporate over time, they don't have staying power; you may want to reapply during the day. Also, the pigments are concentrated, so the color you see in

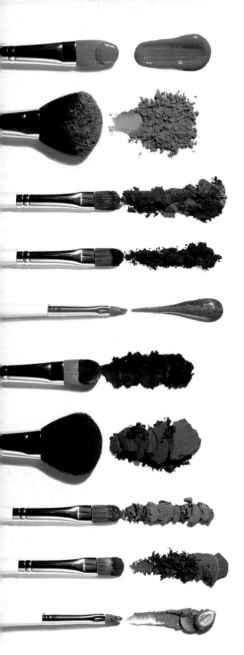

the tube or pot will be a lot more intense than what you actually see on your cheeks. Test the color and consistency on the back of your hand before buying.

Application: Blend in with your fingers. Skip sponges and brushes when it comes to gels.

Creams give cheeks a radiant glow, and some double nicely as eye or lip color. They are emollient and best for drier skins.

Application: Using a sponge for extra control, apply with light, feathery strokes until you achieve the perfect hue. Just a few easy dabs will do.

Powder blush is the most popular and long-lasting form. Easy does it! Powders are more intense in color, and a little goes a long way. If you go too far, gently dab the area with a sponge to remove some color, or dust with a bit of loose or pressed powder to soften the color.

Application: Use a professional blush brush that is medium full for controlled blending. (Toss the brush that comes with the compact. It's usually too small and angular to blend well and can make blush look streaky.)

Get That Glow

Bronzer A favorite product of many top models, a bronzer can give your skin a natural, healthy and dewy glow. Select a shade just a hint deeper than your skin color. If your skin is light, take care to select a shade that won't turn orange on you. Light to dark, you'll find a bevy of colors and consistencies to choose from. A sweep of bronzer on bare skin is alluring. The sheerest formulations take the place of foundation beautifully. Keep it light for day and intensify for evening. Creams and liquids make magic on bare arms, shoulders, back and legs. A beauty tip we learned from our models: Add a bit of bronzer around the hairline and jaw-lines and chin for a sun-kissed look.

Highlighter Highlighters bring "forward" the areas you want to accentuate—such as cheekbones, the bridge of your nose, under the arch of your brows and jawbone. Unlike a bronzer, a highlighter needs more precision in applying: Add it on just the bony area you want to accentuate. Blend and smooth with a finger or sponge.

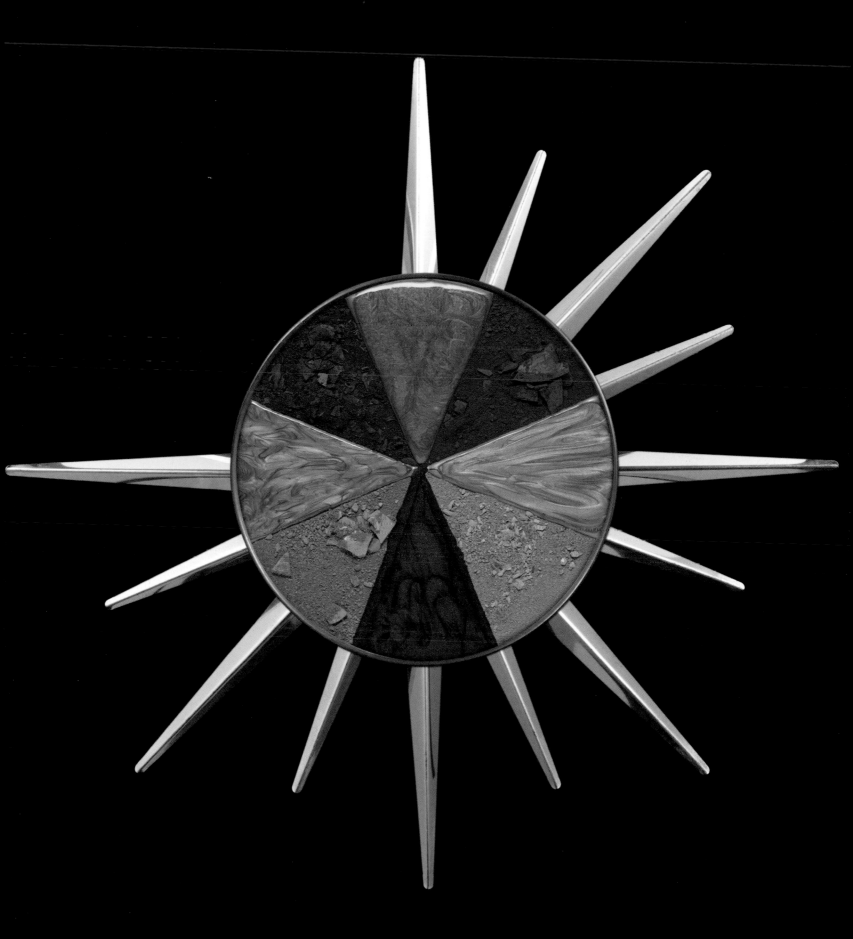

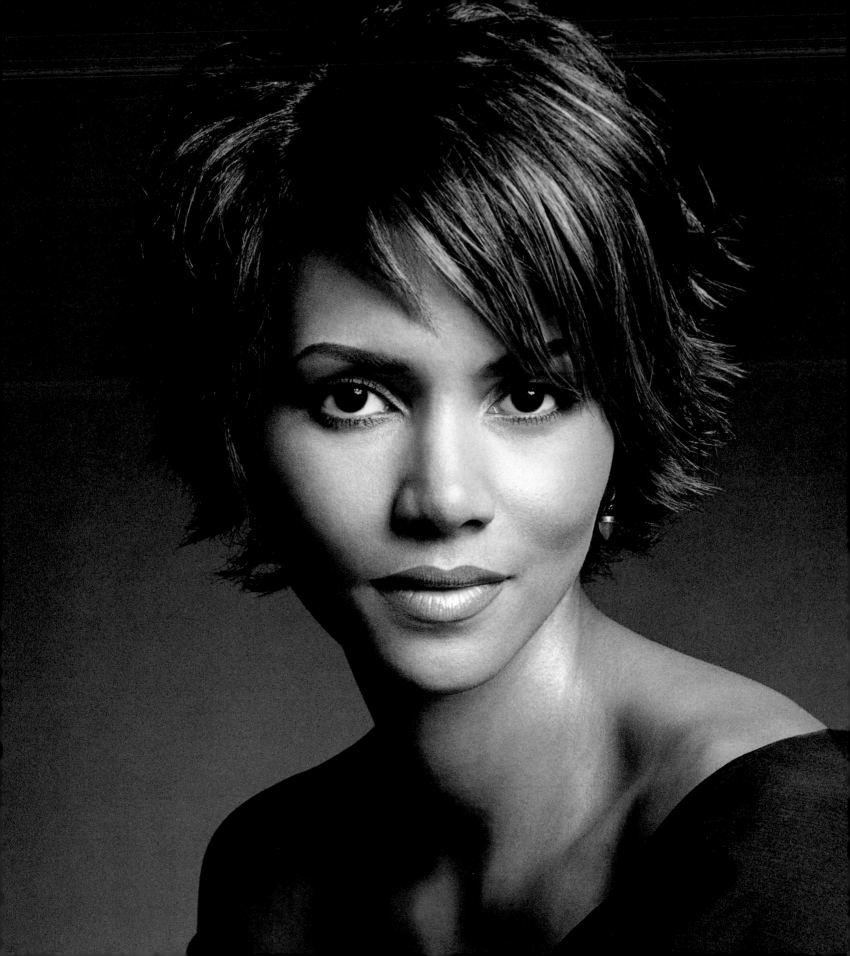

Contouring: Sculpting Your Look

Contouring is the makeup trick to master. Its principles are simple, but you'll need practice to become an expert at it. Basically, contouring involves working with shades a bit lighter and a little darker than your skin color to sculpt and define (and, some makeup pros say, change) the look of your features. And it's all very subtle. Work with the texture that's easiest for you to handle—liquid, stick, cream or powder. Many of the top makeup artists contour with foundation and recommend buying two additional shades, one lighter and one darker. Contouring creates an optical illusion and can make features appear fuller or narrower. Makeup artists literally "sculpt" and change features for photography and film. They recommend that you carefully study your features and decide what you want to amplify or tone down. During the day, use contouring shades ever-so sparingly. If you're spending the evening bathed in candlelight, you can intensify.

Four Contouring Tricks to Try at Home

Here are four easy ways to start having fun with contouring:

1. Eyes on the Prize

If you have droopy eyelids or puffy eyes, create the illusion of bright-eyed vitality by using neutrals like earth, coffee or charcoal to create a smoky eye. Apply the darker neutral shade all over the lid and blend it in to camouflage the droop. Use a lighter shade such as gold or butternut on the brow bone and blend, blend, blend until the shadow almost disappears, but your eyes appear natural and lifted. Finish by curling lashes and applying two coats of black volumizing mascara to top lashes only.

2. The Nose Knows

To define your nose, apply the darker shade along the sides, avoiding the middle. With a finger or a very narrow brush, add the lighter shade down the center of the nose and blend until there's no line of demarcation.

3. Getting Cheeky With It

Here's how to highlight your cheekbones or create the illusion of more prominent ones: Use a lighter foundation on the mound of your cheek and a sweep of the darker shade just under the bone. Blend well. Then using a fluffy blush brush, apply blush to the mound of your cheekbone and up to the hairline, and blend well. Stripey cheeks—not good!

4. Chin Up

Soften the appearance of a double chin by blending your deeper contour shade onto the area just underneath the chin and jawline, from left to right.

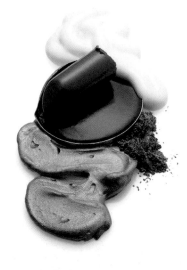

Eyebrows:
How to Achieve the Perfect Shape

Well-groomed eyebrows open up the eye and frame the face. Our best advice: Find an eyebrow pro in your area to shape yours, and every other day or so tweeze any new growth. You can keep the perfect shape for a month. When you can't make it to the salon, follow these simple steps to get your best brows.

Three Easy Steps

Step 1: Assess. Whether you like full, luxuriant brows or thin, exquisite arched ones, you can get the perfect shape with or without a professional's hand. Remember, the best brows always follow their natural shape. With your natural brow as a guide, use an eyeliner pencil to draw the shape you want. Don't focus too much on trends. Work with a brow shape that flatters your face. Practicing with a pencil, you can decide on the length, shape and arch that frame your eyes best before removing a hair.

Step 2: Shape. Make sure you have the basic tools: tweezers, cuticle scissors, a clear mascara, a white eye pencil, an eyebrow pencil or powder and a small brow brush. Looking into a magnifying mirror, use clear mascara to brush brows upward. Let them dry so that the hairs are easier

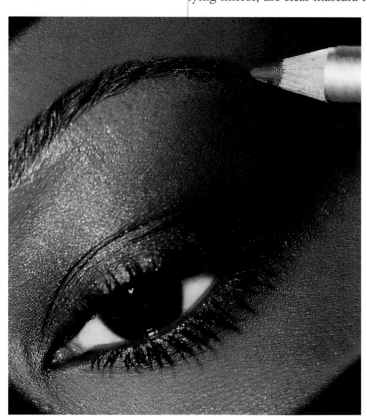

to shape. With the cuticle scissors, trim longer hairs above the upper brow line outside the desired shape. Then apply white pencil to hairs below the brow that need to be removed. Tweeze hairs by pulling in the direction they grow—one hair at a time so the shape of your brows is precise and just right. Repeat on your other brow. Finally, brush your brows with clear mascara again to be sure you haven't missed any hairs.

Step 3: Define. Look in the mirror. Are there any sparse areas? If you've gone too far and the head of the brow, which is near your nose, looks overplucked or the tail too thin, fill the spaces with powder or pencil, one stroke at a time for the most natural look. Powder calls for the lightest hand. After filling brows in, blend with a small brow brush. To keep eyebrows looking great, makeup artists and models set them upward with clear mascara. Avoid using black pencil or powders. Black brows look harsh and artificial. A dark-brown shade looks natural.

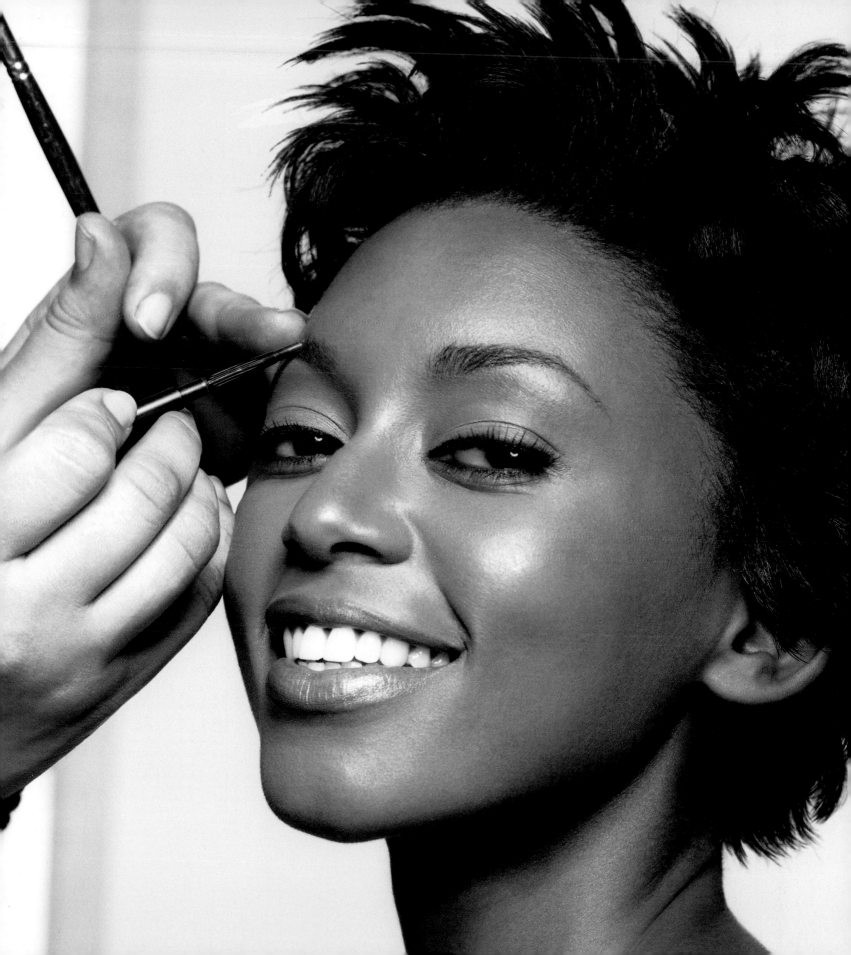

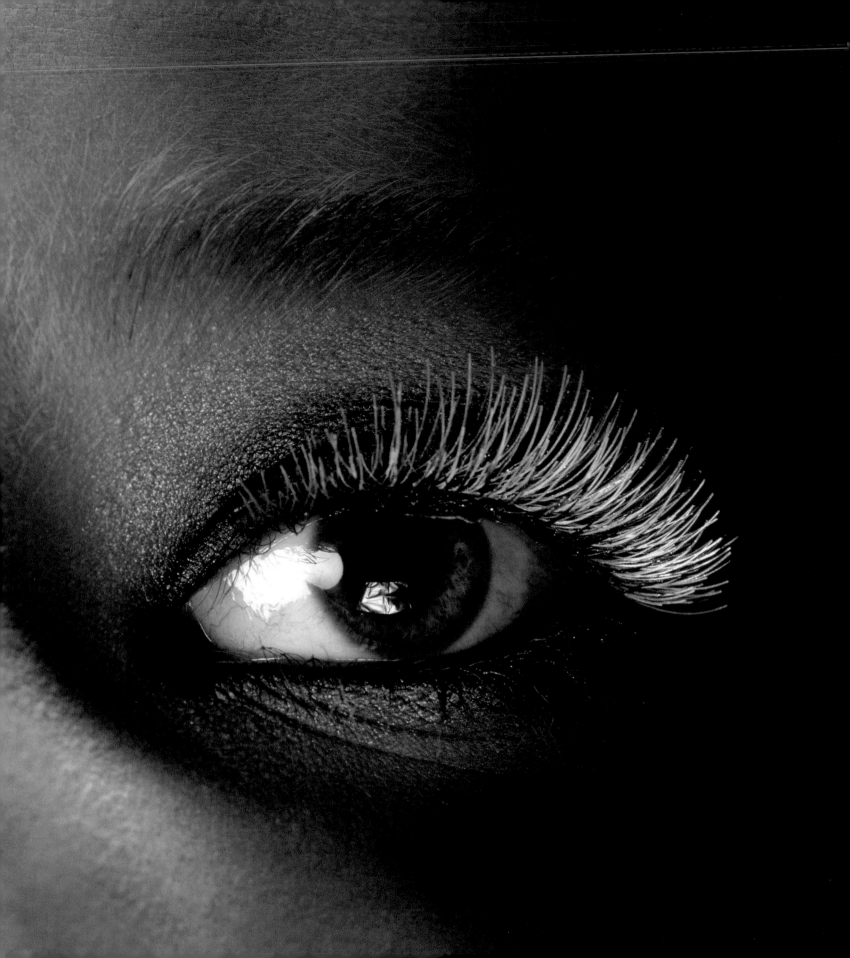

Metallic shadows look great on our skin. Look for warm, metallic neutrals with subtle shimmer to add a spark to your eyes.

Concealer not only covers dark circles, but it also works as a great eye-shadow base. Dab a tiny amount around the entire eye, and blend well to help shadow stay put.

Eyes: Glamorize Your Gaze

Behold the power of your eyes. Take the best care of them with regular visits to an ophthalmologist. And you can learn how to make the most of your most expressive feature with makeup. Eye makeup—shimmery, matte, deep or dramatic—help telegraph your emotions in Technicolor! Making up the eyes is easy when you follow this advice from our experts.

Shadow 101

Keep it simple when it comes to making up your eyes. The most you'll ever need are three shades: a medium tone for your lids, a darker one for the crease under your brow bone and a lighter shade for highlighting just under the arch of your brow. A pretty neutral shade (any warm hue from golden taupe to coffee) on your lids is enough for a quick bit of polish. At times you'll want to play; go ahead and experiment with the palette of colors available today.

Making Eyes

No time for complicated blending and shading? Simply blend a powder, cream or liquid eye shadow from the lash line to the crease. Today's eye is less contoured and dramatic—especially for daytime. You can crank up the glam by creating a thin line of dark brown or black eyeliner along the top lash line and sweeping on volumizing mascara.

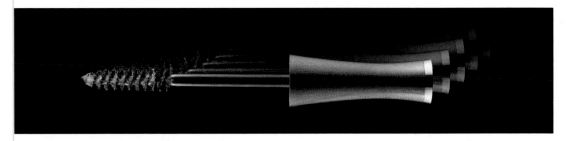

Liquid Liner Cheat Sheet

Nothing says glamour quite like liquid liner. Here's how to master the art of the line in two simple steps. Any expert will tell you that with these moves, practice makes perfect.

Step 1: Look into a magnifying mirror and place the middle finger of your left hand on the outer corner of your left eye and give the area a gentle tug: This will lengthen your eyelid, making application a snap.

Step 2: Using your right hand, hold the brush between your thumb and forefinger. Now place it at the inner corner of your eye and slowly sweep the brush across your lid as close as possible to lashes, ending just past your lash line. The result: a sleek smooth sweep from start to finish.

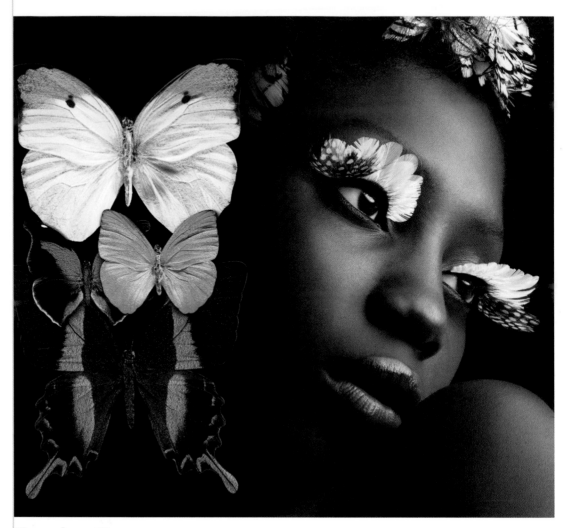

Evening Eyes

Sundown is a time for experimenting with diva-dramatic eyes. First, prevent late-night creasing by blending a dot of foundation across lid, closing your eyes and setting with loose powder. Next, get smoky by applying a color with impact, such as charcoal, navy, eggplant or burgundy, from the lash line up to the crease, then sweep a luminous highlighter along brow bone. Finally, line the inner rims of the eye with a black pencil, and accentuate lashes with a coat of black lengthening mascara or fake lashes.

Cat Eyes

The cat eye, popular in the fifties, is back. Here's the easiest way to get the look: Using the finest, thinnest pointy eyeliner brush, dot a thin row of cream or liquid eyeliner along top lash line. Next, blend the dots together to create one solid line. It's sometimes difficult to get this line in one sweep. So, simply connect the small dots along the lash line outward. Then thicken the line slightly just beyond the end of your eye.

Many Black women have two-toned lips. One lip, usually the bottom, may be lighter than the other. Go with it. Just add gloss and learn to love what the Creator made.

Avoid leaving a "lipstick kiss" on your cocktail glass by discreetly licking the rim before sipping. The wetness will form a barrier, minimizing the transfer of color.

When you want to even out lip color, apply a layer of foundation to lips, then use a lip brush to apply a lipstick in a texture that gives you great coverage. Try any long-lasting shade, and presto—you've got all-in-one-tone lips!

Lips: Your Pretty Pout

Make the most of the shape of your lips, which are one of every person's most unique features. Love them and protect them. Keep lips soft by exfoliating and moist by using nourishing balms every night. Rub your lips with a warm wet washcloth to slough off dry skin, and apply a rich moisturizing balm before going to bed.

Breaking the Color Rules

When it comes to lipstick shades, kick any rules to the curb. We love mixing it up. Chocolate sisters can look fabulous even wearing only the right shades of pink, and the café au lait sisters can easily rock the deepest plums. Thanks to new technology, textures and hues can come on strong or light and sheer. To kick up your glam, experiment with colors and textures. Choose your faves and have fun!

Nude Awakenings

Neutral, natural-looking lips are so alluring. When you're in a rush, just try filling in lips with a neutral lip pencil, swipe on clear gloss and go! This look is sheer, lovely and moisturizing. To add a bit of pizzazz, use a gloss that's a shimmery shade of copper.

Red Hot

Red lips make a classic statement and command attention. Choose cool tones like candy-apple or burgundy, or warm shades like cinnamon or maroon.

Liner Notes

The point of liner is to keep lip color in place, to prevent it from "bleeding." Liner also creates a finished, clean look. Don't consider lining lips in a shade darker than your lips or your lip-

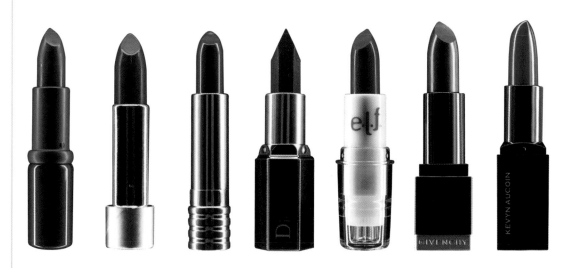

To keep lipstick on your lips and off your teeth, cover your finger in a tissue and hold it inside of your mouth while touching your teeth. Close your lips gently around your finger then pull your finger out of your mouth. The excess color will rub off on the tissue and not on your pearlies.

To ensure that your lipstick doesn't bleed, smear or budge, blend a few dots of foundation around your mouth, outside the lip line before applying lip color. Then set the foundation by brushing on a bit of loose translucent powder. Line your lips and apply your lipstick.

Don't let your eyes compete with your lips. When one is dramatic, go neutral with the other.

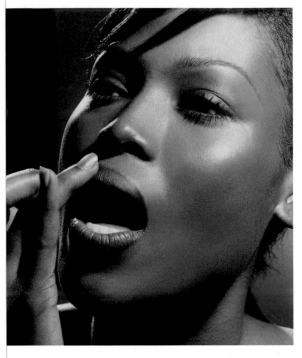

stick—that style was hot back in the day, but now it's passé. Pick a lip-liner pencil that exactly matches your natural lip color when wearing neutral shades of gloss or lipstick or one that's close to any intense lipstick shade you choose.

It's the Balm

To protect your lips from sun or wind damage and to fight flaky, chapped lips, which can also be painful, use the most sumptuous lip balm before applying lipstick or gloss, or just wear balm alone. Tinted balms add a slick of sheer color while keeping lips moisturized. You can even find neutral and tinted balms with sun protection for added benefits.

Lip Lingo

➤ If you want moist lips with an opaque, satin finish, choose cream lipstick.
➤ If you want enduring matte lips with a see-through finish, reach for a lip stain.
➤ For lips that are shiny and sexy, go for lip gloss; be prepared to reapply often.
➤ When you want lips that sparkle, use a metallic lipstick.

Allergy Season Advice

Along with giving you an itchy throat and watery eyes, allergy season can wreak havoc on your makeup. Follow these easy tips to avoid the seasonal dilemmas that pollen can bring.

➤ **Use natural products** found in health-food stores. Doing so will help prevent red, itchy eyes from sensitivity to ingredients in eye makeup.
➤ **After a sneezing session,** clean up an eye makeup mess with a cotton swab. Dab the swab in moisturizer or with a bit of water, and gently wipe the area (no tugging!).
➤ **If you wear foundation,** keep your compact close by. Touch up after blowing your nose.
➤ **Look for a long-wearing foundation.** This formulation can prevent undereye makeup breakup.
➤ **Pull a contouring trick** out of your bag. Apply contour color to the brow bone to offset the look of the swollen, red eyes that are infamous with allergy season.
➤ **Skip eye makeup altogether.** It's OK to sacrifice beauty for your health now and then. Give your eyes a break when you are having a particularly rough day with pollen.

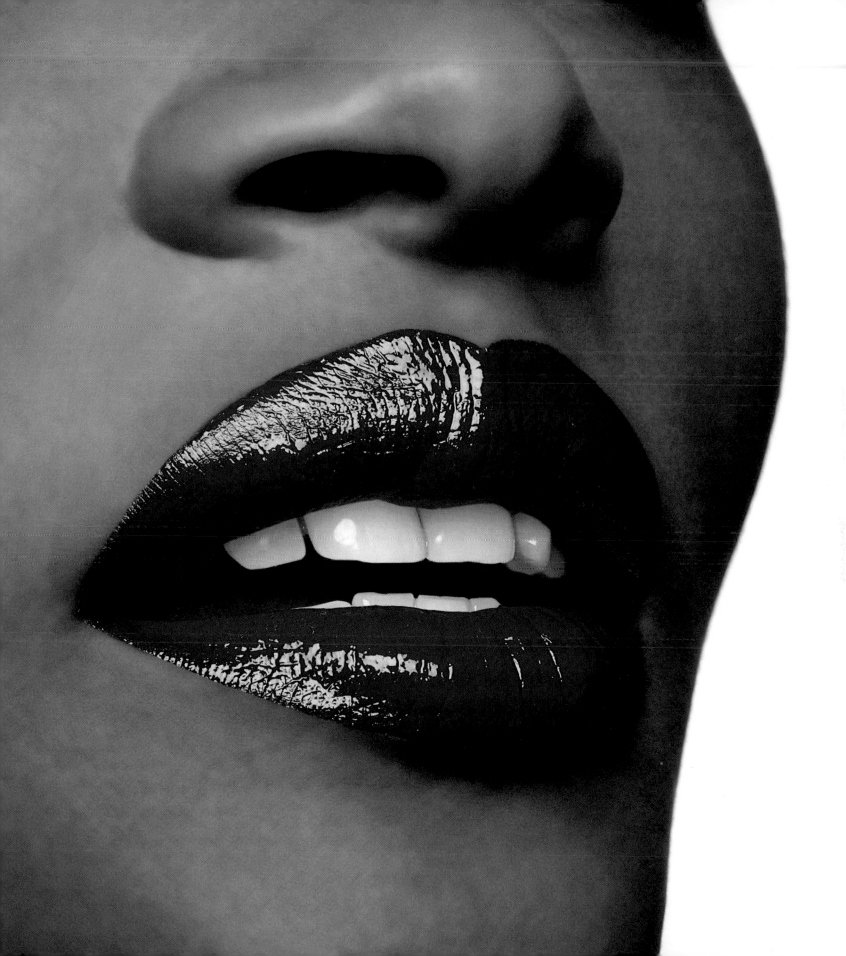

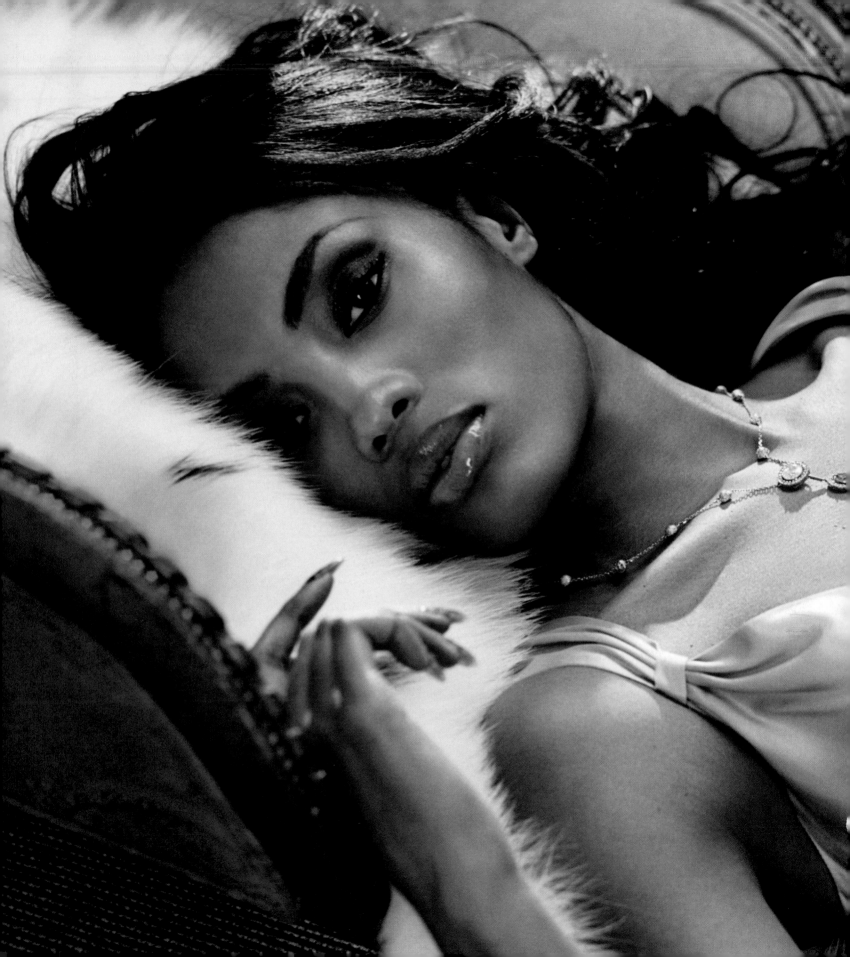

Shelf Life

We all have our favorite beauty products that may last for years. But holding on to makeup too long can breed bacteria and cause skin irritation and breakouts. This chart tells you when it's time to ditch your beauty stash in exchange for new goods.

Foundation

**6–12 months
6 months for liquid and cream foundations**

Extend your foundation's life by using a cotton swab or sponge to apply it. If you use your fingers to apply your makeup, wash your hands with an antibacterial cleanser first. Stick formulations can be kept a bit longer because they often contain more wax. Shave off the top layer periodically to avoid contamination. However, if you notice a change in color, smell or consistency, toss it.

Powder

8 months for compact; 8–12 months for loose powder

Applicators like brushes and powder puffs pose the greatest risk of contamination because they can harbor oily buildup from your skin and airborne bacteria when left uncovered. Toss sponges after each use, and replace powder puffs every 2 to 3 weeks. Wash makeup brushes weekly with baby shampoo and warm water. Let them dry overnight. Damp brushes will cause makeup to streak.

Concealer

4–8 months

If your concealer is in a lipstick form, clean it by occasionally shaving the top layer off. Cover-up used in the eye area should be discarded after six months. And if you're masking acne breakouts, you risk contaminating the product even faster.

Eye Shadow

**3–6 months for liquid;
6–12 months for powder and cream**

Toss your shadow if it gets wet—unless it is formulated for wet applications. Moisture can lead to contamination or ruin the product's performance. Creams will sweat or soften with excessive exposure to heat, so store in a cool place.

Mascara

3 months

Introducing air into a liquid product—which is what happens when you "pump" the wand into the mascara tube—dries out the product, resulting in a less-than-stellar application. If you have to pump to get the product on the brush or are adding water, it's time to let it go.

Lipstick

3 years

Shave a sliver off the top or dip in alcohol weekly to clean. For lip color in pots, remember to swipe the tops with a tissue occasionally to keep them clean. If your lipstick comes in contact with a fever blister or cold sore, throw it away.

Finding Your Look

With the just-right products and regimen for your skin type, you can have the fresh, clear and smooth complexion you want and create the look that makes the most of your unique features. All you need to do is determine what you want and the look that works best for you.

To find your best look, identify your most dominant feature and the one you consider most attractive. Do you think your eyes, lips or cheeks should be highlighted? Decide where you want to attract the most attention, and you've found your focus. Use this general principle as a guide: Light and bright shades make features more prominent; dark shades make features appear to recede. So use lighter, brighter colors to highlight any area and darker, subdued colors to draw attention away from a feature. For example, to bring out the beauty of your eyes, a vibrant or intense lid color will accentuate them. But if you have protruding or hooded eyes, bright and glittering colors will only intensify them. Instead, you'll want to go deeper and wear warm earth tones or shades that will soften and give them allure.

Balancing Act

Our busy lives make it easy to fall into a makeup rut and get stuck with a look that's quick and easy yet the same every day. You can keep it simple and still embrace change. After all, makeup is meant to be enhancing and fun. One day choose an intense lip color, but use a soft blush and a neutral shade on your lids. Here's a simple tip to follow for using color: The key is balance. A neutral look is always gorgeous, but sometimes you want to wake up your makeup with vivid shades. When opting for color, remember that electric brights may look good on the runway but can easily look garish in real time. So go easy.

Intense eyes, soft cheeks, medium lips
Medium eyes, soft cheeks, intense lips
Soft eyes, intense cheeks, medium lips

Try different hues of eyeliners in bronze, plum, copper or green—these colors look great on Black skin tones. Most appear bright in the tube, but eventually dry down into more subtle, attractive colors.

To pick up droopy eyelids, add color to the lids from the outer corner to the center, then blend over the bone. Don't go higher than the crease.

Makeup Tips

➤ Discolored lips can be evened out with lip toners or balancers applied before your lipstick or gloss.
➤ To narrow the nose, apply color along the sides of the nose, but not directly onto the center.
➤ To lift the cheekbones, use your fingers to locate your cheekbones, then brush on a few sweeps of shadow in a diagonal direction toward the top of the ear at the hollow of your cheeks. The result is softer if you apply the shadow in layers.
➤ To camouflage a double chin, shade the area just below the chin, right under the jawline, but not on the neck. Move the brush from left to right.
➤ To define the jawline, brush the color directly under the bone from the ear to the chin.
➤ To highlight your cheekbones, use color high on the cheek and feather color outward toward the upper ear.
➤ Line your lips in a shade that matches your lipstick to help create a defined, gorgeous mouth.

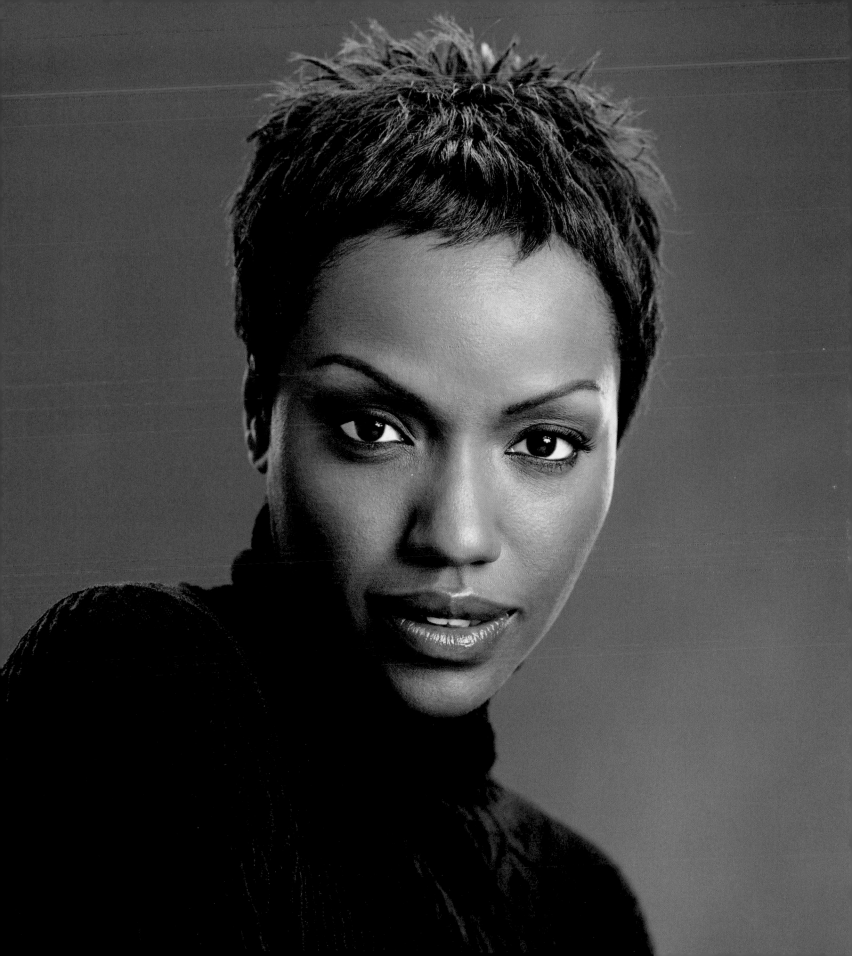

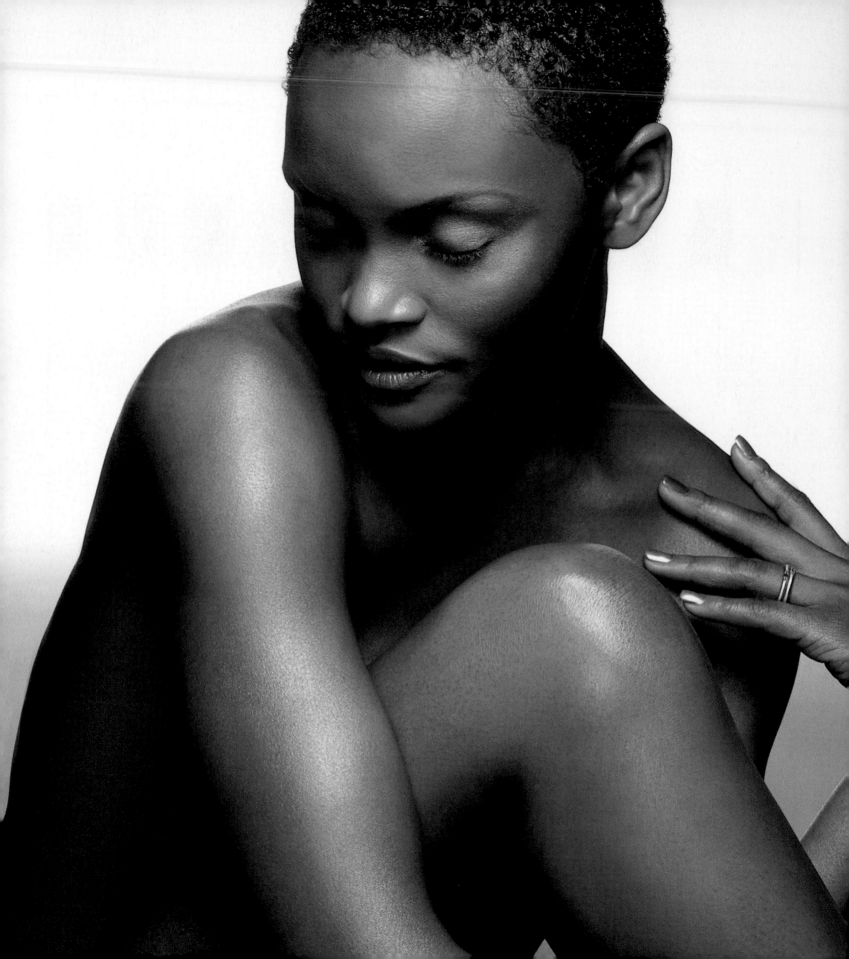

Your Best
Body

The body is a miracle, a gift from the Creator to be cherished and cared for all the days of our lives. Each of us is a divine original. We shouldn't compare ourselves to the unrealistic ideal the media force-feeds us. Lavish your body with the best care around. It's important to love yourself from head to toe and inside out.

Condition with avocados. The oil easily penetrates the skin, making it an ideal ingredient for moisturizing body treatments.

Switch to soy. As an ingredient in skin care products, soy extract softens and smoothes skin, replenishes moisture, helps brighten dark spots and is a proven antioxidant.

Peel a pomegranate. The seeds are excellent for body buffing, and the fruit provides a mild astringent with antioxidant properties.

Get into grapes. Red, green or purple as grapeseed extract in some products can fight free radicals and calm the skin.

Carrot, celery and beet juice cleanse the liver and intestines, which will help clear up the complexion.

Pay Attention to Nutrition

To look great on the outside you must take care of your body from the inside, so eating healthy food is an important part of the beauty process. Providing your body with the proper nutrients will help ensure healthy vibrant skin. Minimize or eliminate fatty meat, white flour, sugar, processed foods and full-fat dairy products. Instead, opt for naturally bright-colored fruits and vegetables (think orange, green and yellow), and increase your share of nuts, olive oil and wild, not farm-raised, fish. Replace dairy with soy products and low-fat yogurt.

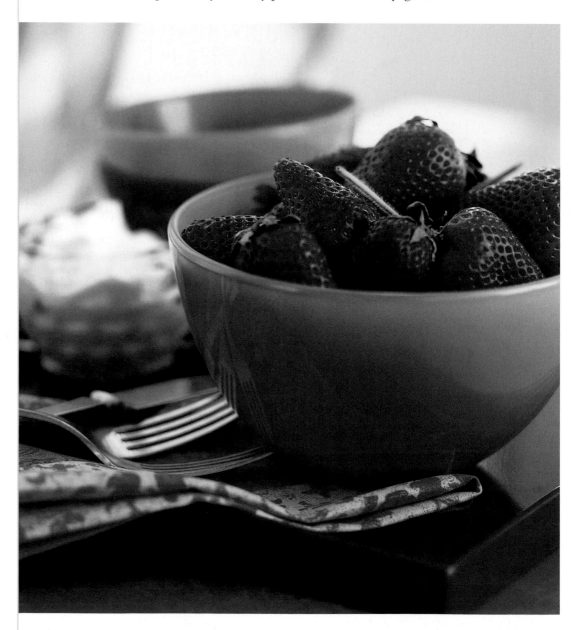

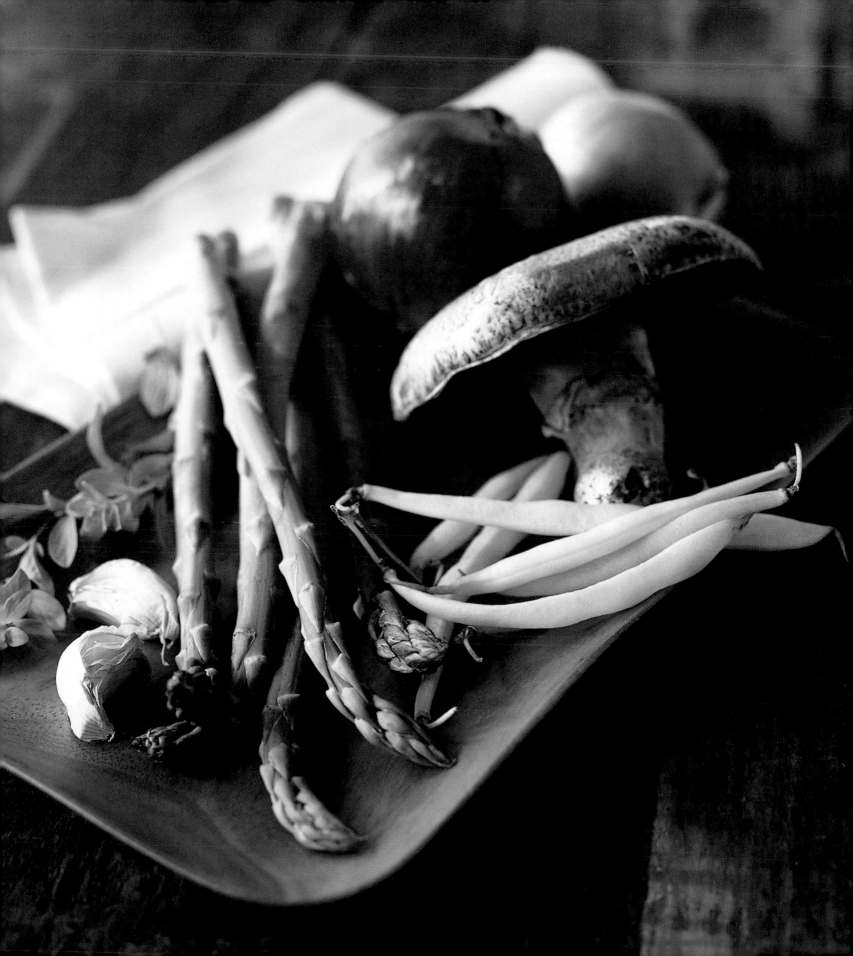

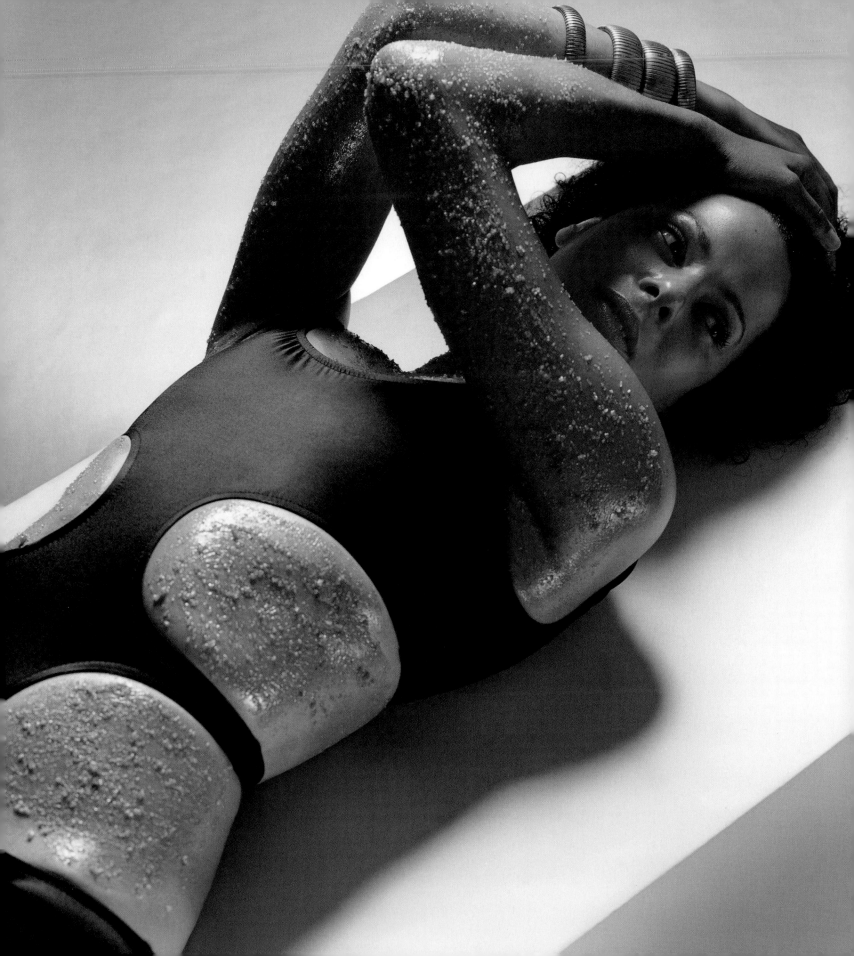

Body Beauty Basics

The best overall skin-care regimen is based on simplicity. You don't need dozens of expensive products. Just remember to follow three easy steps to keep your body beautiful and skin glowing.

1. Cleanse. Start your body-care regime with a warm bath or shower to open pores and release some of the impurities built up on the skin's surface. Use a fragrant body wash, or if you have time, soak in therapeutic mineral salts.

2. Exfoliate. Keep skin soft, supple and glowing by using a salt- or sugar-based body scrub or a loofah with a hydrating shower gel. Both techniques help purge built-up layers of dead skin, making room for your natural luster to shine through. You can use loofahs and shower gels daily, but turn to body scrubs no more than twice a week as they tend to have a drying effect. Remember not to scrub too aggressively, or you'll wind up with raw, irritated skin.

3. Hydrate. To keep skin moist, follow exfoliation with an emollient-rich moisturizer like shea butter. Look for lotions containing glycerin, an ingredient that keeps skin moist longer. To seal in moisture, apply the body cream, oil or lotion to slightly damp skin. And remember to hydrate your skin from the inside out by drinking at least eight glasses of water each day.

Try exfoliating with a skin brush, which can be found at body-care stores. After a shower, brush dry skin in an upward motion using circular strokes across the buttocks, thighs, legs and knees. This will remove dead skin and stimulate collagen production, which leaves skin firm and glowing.

Add to your basic body cream a mixture of white tea (a great source of antioxidants) and four drops of a relaxing essential oil like sage, which helps soothe and moisturize.

Before heading outdoors, protect your skin with sunscreen that has an SPF of 15 or higher. Now beauty products such as foundations, lotions and lip gloss also contain SPF protection.

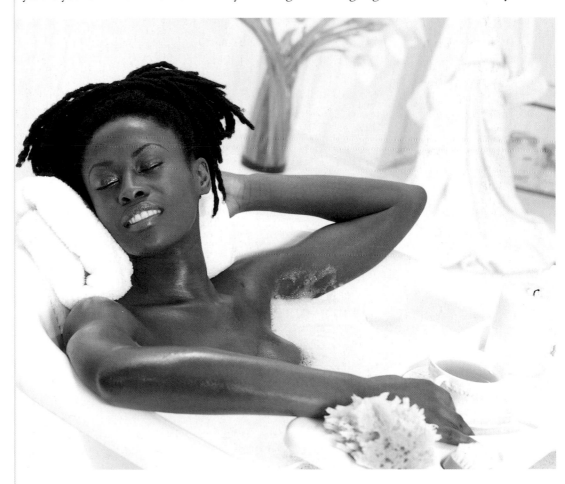

A Whiter, Brighter Smile

Brushing and flossing at least twice a day keeps gums healthy and teeth cavity-free, but following the basics isn't always enough to keep teeth their whitest and brightest. Whether you are seeking professional help for a take-home custom bleaching plan or want less-expensive, over-the-counter whitening systems, several options can help you get a stand-out smile.

In-Office Bleaching

How It Works: Using an airbrush-type tool, a dental professional blasts your teeth with a bleaching solution to remove layers of darkened color.

Pro: You can do the procedure on your lunch hour.

Cons: It costs anywhere from $600 and up, plus you may feel sensitivity to cold and warm foods after the procedure.

Dentist-Prescribed Bleaching Tray

How It Works: A prescribed bleaching gel made of carbomide peroxide is squeezed into a custom-made vinyl template of your teeth for you to wear at home for two or more hours each day over about two weeks.

Pros: This option costs less than regular visits to your dentist, and it can be done at home after your initial in-office consultation.

Con: Sensitivity to cold and warm foods may occur after two to three weeks.

Over-the-Counter Bleaching Products

How They Work: Typically offered in the form of bleaching toothpaste or coated bleaching strips, these products are used twice a day for about two weeks to brighten teeth.

Pros: You can do this technique at home, at a fraction of the cost of anything the dentist prescribes.

Con: At-home bleaching products only produce minimum results—don't expect drastic changes.

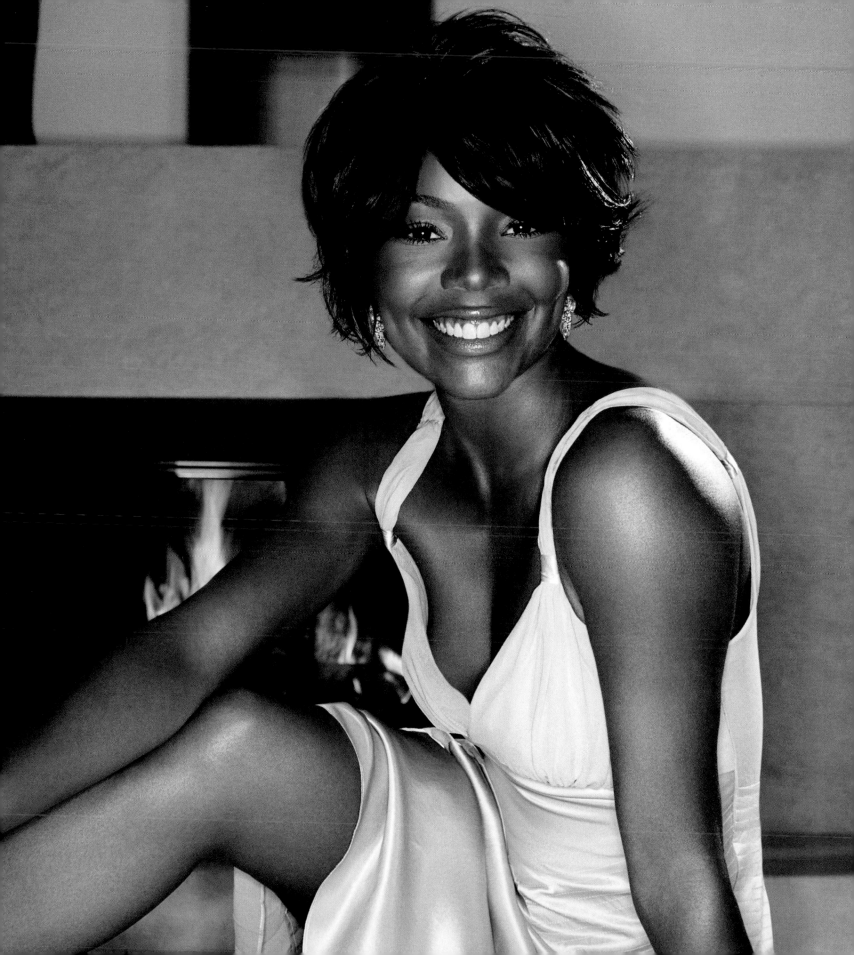

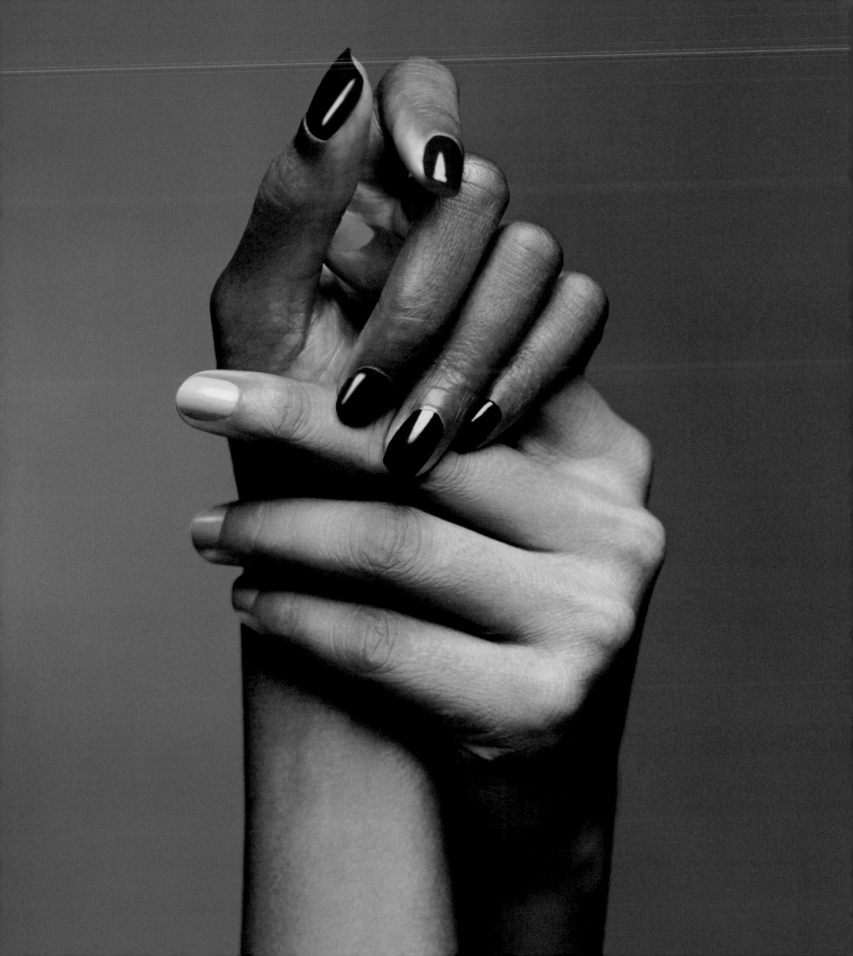

Make sure to keep hands and cuticles moisturized throughout the day. Consider using an ultrahydrating lotion with an SPF to fight dryness and ward off sun-rays.

When polishing, try lighter colors like beige or white to camouflage imperfect nails.

A Winning Hand

Beautifully manicured hands speak volumes about a woman—people notice your hands. That's why a weekly pampering plan focused on your hands and nails is a must on your to-do list. Whether your nails need protection against breakage, peeling and splitting or just require an extra boost of moisture, a few simple steps can make your hands look healthy and lovely in no time flat.

Protect

Increase your calcium intake, which can help prevent chipping and peeling and provide a protective shield. Eat leafy green vegetables, low-fat dairy products and hijiki (a calcium-packed sea vegetable served at Japanese restaurants), and take a calcium supplement. Using nail products containing calcium pantothenate, protein and vitamin E can also strengthen nails. Remember to wear cotton-lined rubber gloves when doing chores and never to use your nails as tools. Apply cuticle oil at night to help fortify nails.

Grow

After you've protected your nails, coat them with strengtheners that contain vitamins A, C and E to help them grow. Add to your diet some iron, folic acid, zinc and protein, which are all beneficial nutrients for healthy nails, along with a B vitamin supplement like biotin, which is proven to improve brittle nails.

The Perfect Pointers: At-Home Manicure

➤ **Soften.** Soak nails in warm water. This first step helps soften the cuticles.
➤ **Shape.** Use a nail file with a grid between 140 and 200 (hard-grid nail files do too much damage to the nail bed) to shape the nail. A soft almond or square shape gives nails an elegant look and makes nails less prone to breakage.
➤ **Push.** Use an orangewood stick to push cuticles back. Never cut them!
➤ **Polish.** Apply a base coat, two coats of nail color and a top coat to seal color. Clean up overage with a cotton swab or orangewood stick wrapped in cotton.

Wake Up With Soft Hands

Before bedtime, try this soothing, smoothing treatment.
➤ **Lubricate** cuticles with vitamin E, jojoba or your favorite oil.
➤ **Massage** hands with warm water.
➤ **Apply** an exfoliating treatment.
➤ **Pat** hands dry.
➤ **Put** another drop of oil on each nail.
➤ **Apply** shea butter on hands to hydrate and cover with cotton gloves—then sleep tight!

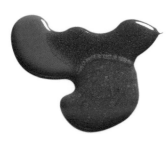

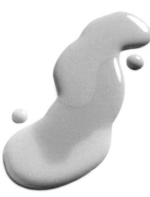

Pamper

Whether you get a professional manicure or do it at home, polished nails show you are "hands on" when it comes to beauty. In addition to basic nail filing and polishing, professional manicures incorporate exfoliation, intense moisturizing, paraffin dips and cuticle treatments. But at-home care can be just as good.

Nail Rx

Your hands are exposed to the elements throughout the day, which can cause dry skin and brittle nails if you don't care for them. Here are three ways to combat damaged nails.

Mix and massage. Combine a drop of cuticle oil with a mild exfoliator, and lightly massage into the nail bed; add conditioning balm if cuticles are damaged to accelerate healing. Or, get more mileage out of keratin-based hair conditioner by using it as a nail moisturizer.

Cure cuticles. Hydrate cuticles and nails by mixing a teaspoon each of sweet almond, jojoba and vitamin E oils, then massaging into hands and nails nightly. You can also hydrate nails by eating a diet enriched in essential fatty acids, which are found in sardines, salmon, green leafy vegetables and walnuts.

Prevent fungus. Nail extensions—such as acrylic or tips—can be a manicure miracle with one major obstacle: fungus, which grows when moisture gets caught between artificial nails and the natural nail bed, leaving a moldy residue. Fungus also rears its ugly head when your nails are exposed to instruments that have not been properly cleaned. The best way to prevent that situation: BYOT—bring your own tools (file, buffer, cuticle remover, nail clipper and orangewood stick) to the nail salon.

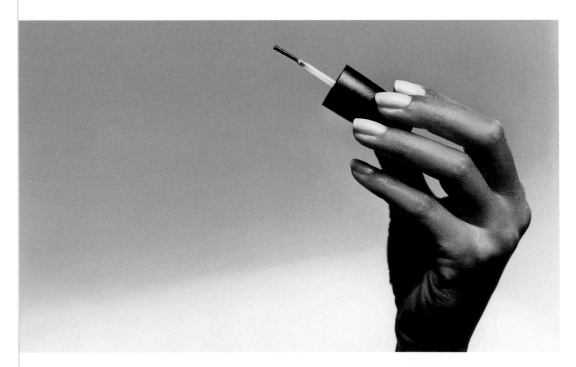

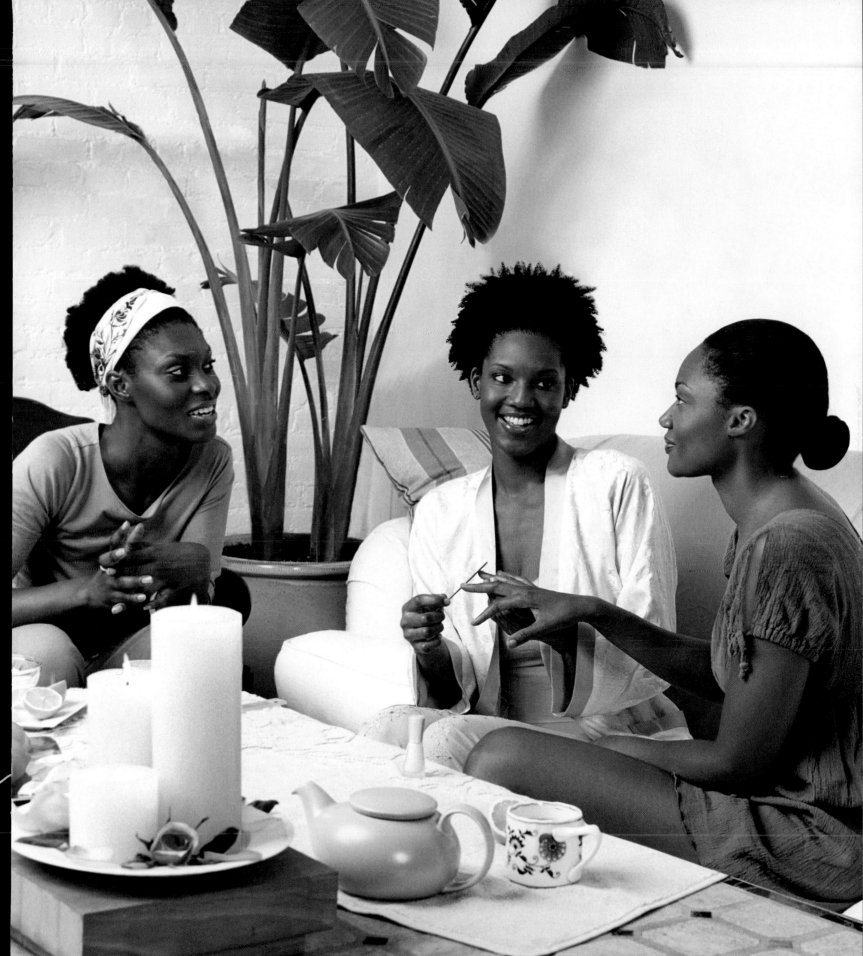

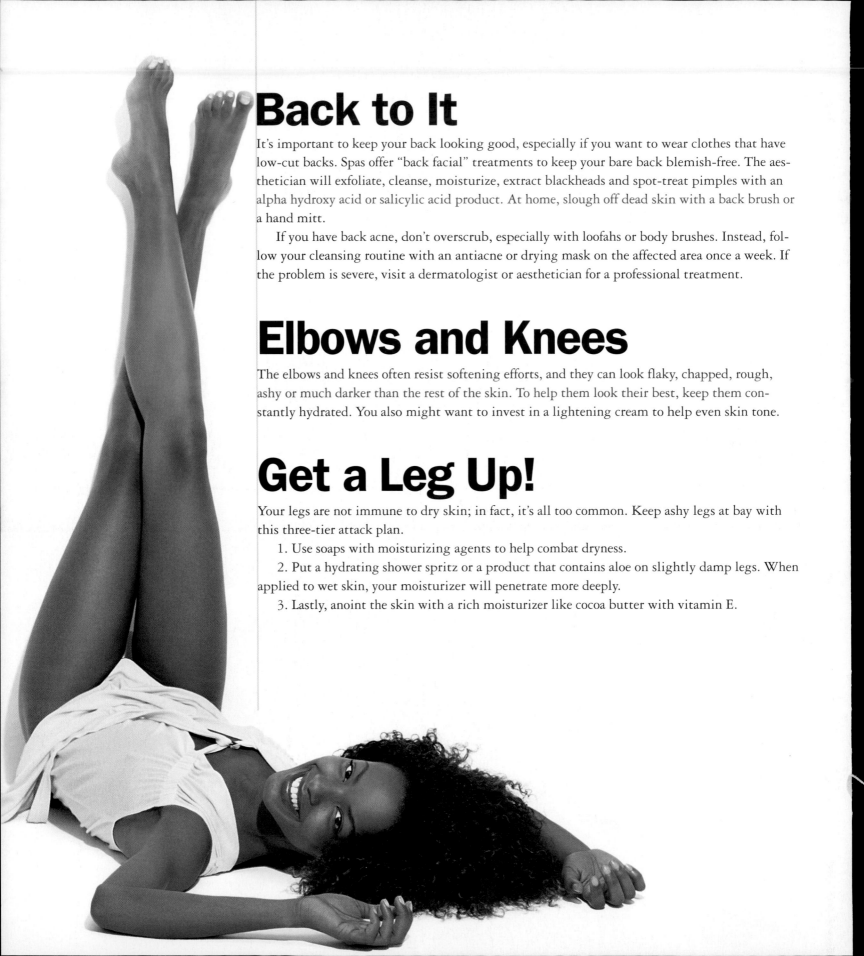

Back to It

It's important to keep your back looking good, especially if you want to wear clothes that have low-cut backs. Spas offer "back facial" treatments to keep your bare back blemish-free. The aesthetician will exfoliate, cleanse, moisturize, extract blackheads and spot-treat pimples with an alpha hydroxy acid or salicylic acid product. At home, slough off dead skin with a back brush or a hand mitt.

If you have back acne, don't overscrub, especially with loofahs or body brushes. Instead, follow your cleansing routine with an antiacne or drying mask on the affected area once a week. If the problem is severe, visit a dermatologist or aesthetician for a professional treatment.

Elbows and Knees

The elbows and knees often resist softening efforts, and they can look flaky, chapped, rough, ashy or much darker than the rest of the skin. To help them look their best, keep them constantly hydrated. You also might want to invest in a lightening cream to help even skin tone.

Get a Leg Up!

Your legs are not immune to dry skin; in fact, it's all too common. Keep ashy legs at bay with this three-tier attack plan.

1. Use soaps with moisturizing agents to help combat dryness.

2. Put a hydrating shower spritz or a product that contains aloe on slightly damp legs. When applied to wet skin, your moisturizer will penetrate more deeply.

3. Lastly, anoint the skin with a rich moisturizer like cocoa butter with vitamin E.

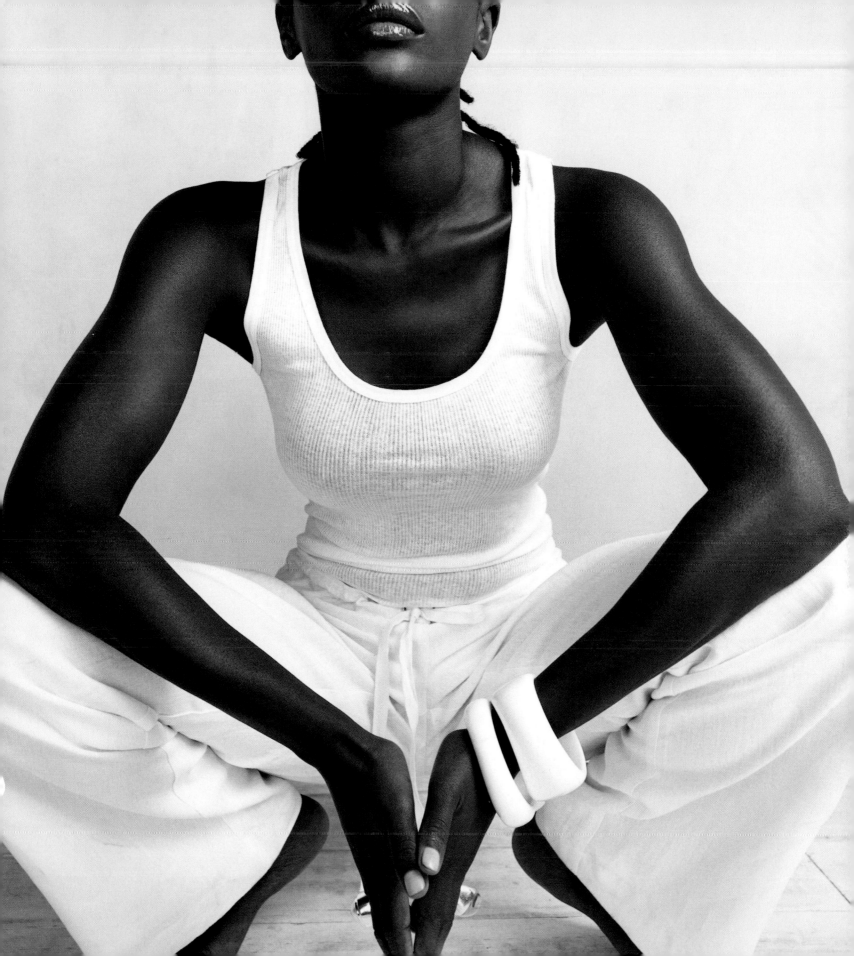

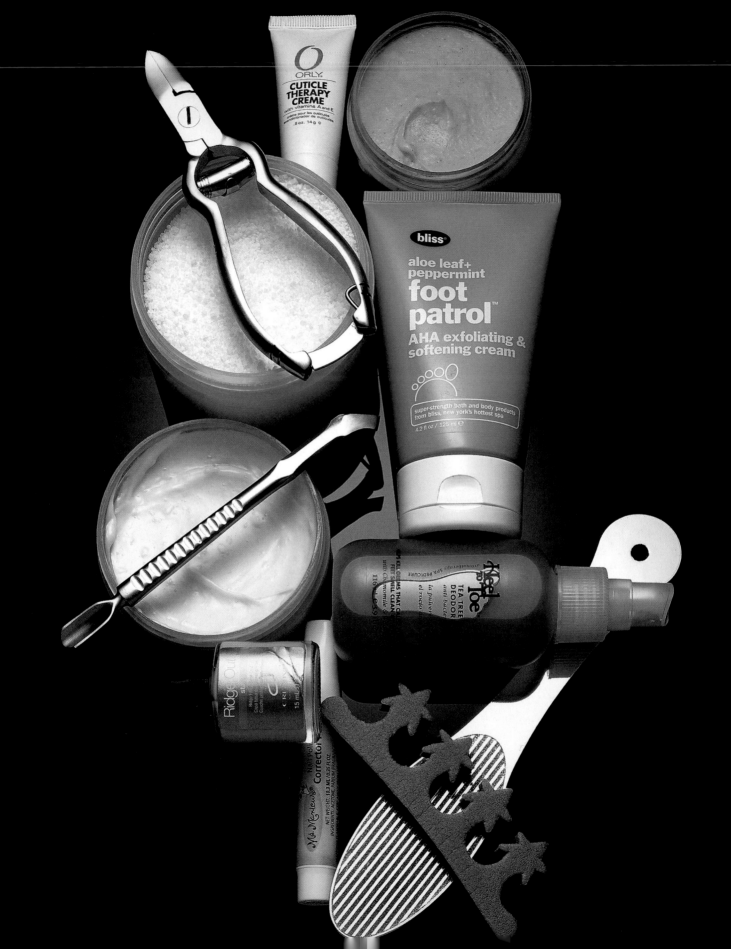

Toe to Toe

Put your best foot forward with regular pedicures—done either by a professional or at home. With proper care, your feet will always be made for showing off your newest shoes.

5 Steps to a Soleful Experience: At-Home Pedicure

1. Prep

First, gather what you will need:

A basin
A toenail clipper
Cuticle oil
A nail file
An orangewood stick
A pumice stone
A towel
Two plastic bags
Toe separators
Cotton
Nail-polish remover
Top and base coats
Polish

Next, wipe off old polish with an acetone-based remover to lift oil and any residue from the nail plate.

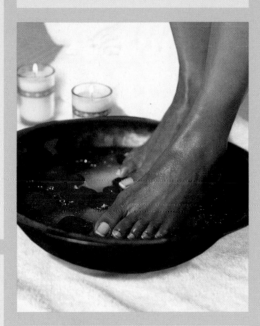

2. Soak

Immerse your feet in liquid to soften dead skin, making it easier to remove. Create your own luxurious pedicure soak by adding 8 to 10 cups of liquid or powdered milk and 10 drops of lavender oil to your foot tub. The lactic acid in milk softens feet faster than water does, while the soothing therapeutic lavender relaxes and calms. Or, try filling the basin with warm water and crushed lemons to cleanse and help dissipate nail discoloration. Then, add one or more of the following: fresh chopped oregano, lemongrass or thyme to combat fungus and aloe to moisturize.

3. Scrub

Remove dead skin by scrubbing it away. Then use a pumice stone. This is the absolute best way to remove calluses—much more gentle than cutting them away. Start by mixing your own scrub: Combine Epsom salt with scented oils, or mix rice and oat flour to exfoliate; dried ginger or mustard seed work to improve circulation; and a few drops of essential oil add extra moisture.

4. Shape

Tidy up the nail bed by pushing back cuticles instead of cutting them. Decrease your risk of getting ingrown nails by avoiding clippers or cuticle cutters on the sides of the toenails. Clip nails straight across, leaving a thin white edge, then file nails straight across.

5. Polish

Slip your toes into toe separators, and remove any pedicure product residue with cotton and polish remover. Then apply a base coat. Now you are ready for polish. Choose your color and begin with a thin stroke of polish in the middle of the nail, then brush outward to cover the sides. Apply a second coat. Finish with top coat for shine and to seal color. Allow at least an hour for your nails to dry.

Go Bare: A Guide to Hair Removal

From eyebrows and underarms to bikini lines, hair removal is a vital part of the grooming process. Today, you can choose from a variety of hair removal methods to get precisely shaped brows and hairless legs.

Shaving

➤ **What It Is:** Using a razor, shave slowly in the direction of the hair growth, after bathing.

➤ **How It Works:** The heat and water opens pores and softens hair, allowing for a closer shave. To reduce the chance of ingrown hairs, exfoliate skin in the area the day before shaving. Razors start at about $5.

➤ **Best Use:** Underarms, stomach and the bikini area are the best targets for your shaving routine. Caution: Excessive shaving can darken the skin.

Tweezing

➤ **What It Is:** Pulling out hair with tweezers is as precise as it comes and is best for quick clean-ups or small areas of hair.

➤ **How It Works:** Before tweezing eyebrows, clean your brow with a little witch hazel, then pluck hair in the direction of growth. To round off your efforts, brush brows upward and trim excess hair with small grooming scissors for a nice neat effect. Professional tweezing runs about $10 to $50.

➤ **Best Use:** Tweezing is best done only on your eyebrows.

Depilatories

➤ **What They Are:** Chemical solutions that dissolve the hair, depilatories are offered in lotion, foam or cream formulas.

➤ **How They Work:** This method involves smoothing the depilatory onto clean, dry skin, waiting the allotted specified time, and wiping the area with a warm washcloth. Opt for a fast-acting formula you can rinse off in the shower. Products cost $5 to $90.

➤ **Best Use:** Depilatories are convenient for your face, underarms, arms, stomach and bikini area.

At-Home Waxing

Want to try waxing at home? Pick up a kit at your local drugstore, and follow these simple instructions. Try waxing your legs, since they are easy for you to reach. Here's how:

➤ **Prep dry skin with baby powder.** This step helps the wax adhere to the hair, as well as absorb moisture.

➤ **Test first.** To avoid an allergic reaction, try out a dab of wax on your hand first, then apply a small 3–4-inch section of wax in the direction of the hair growth. (As you gain experience, you can work with larger sections.)

➤ **Apply a muslin strip.** Available with most at-home kits, the strip gets placed over the wax. Once the wax has cooled, hold skin taut with one hand and use the other to pull the strip away from your skin in the opposite direction of the hair growth.

➤ **Tip:** Our skin tends to be more sensitive the week before our periods, so skip waxing during this time of the month.

➤ **Tip:** After shaving or waxing, remember to replenish moisture to your skin.

Waxing

➤ **What It Is:** Warm wax is used to catch and pull the hair by the root.

➤ **How It Works:** The wax is spread onto the skin where hair exists. Next, a muslin strip is placed on top of the wax, allowed to cool, then pulled off in the opposite direction of hair growth. To maximize results, it's best to wax areas where hair is a quarter of an inch thick. Exfoliating between waxing sessions lessens the chance of ingrown hairs, but if you have sensitive skin, don't scrub prior to a waxing session because the dead skin can actually act as a buffer against irritation. Salons and spas offer waxing services, but you can also do it at home yourself. Waxing starts at about $5 for upper lip or eyebrows.

➤ **Best Use:** Your face, underarms, arms, stomach and bikini area are all appropriate spots for waxing.

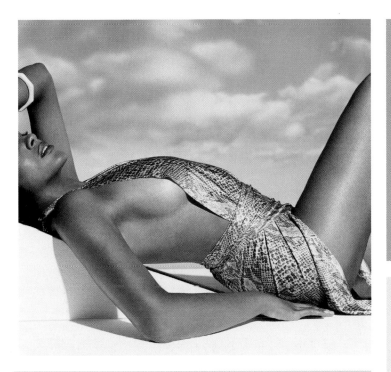

Sugaring

➤ **What It Is:** The ancient practice of sugaring—which is a gel-like formula created from sugar, lemon and water—is an alternative to waxing and is best for sensitive skin.

➤ **How It Works:** An aesthetician applies the sugar solution to the area designated for hair removal in the same way as hot wax. But unlike wax, sugar does not stick to skin, so it's less irritating. Cost starts at $10 for facial hair and more for other parts of the body.

➤ **Best Use:** Your face, underarms, arms, stomach, bikini area and legs can all benefit from sugaring.

Threading

➤ **What It Is:** Threading is a centuries-old Middle Eastern practice that uses sewing thread to remove hair.

➤ **How It Works:** The thread is quickly wound around individual hairs, twisted and used to pull hair out from the follicle. This highly precise method is a lot easier on the skin than waxing. You can't do this method at home. Threading starts at $5.

➤ **Best Use:** Threading is done to remove hair on your face (eyebrows and chin areas).

Electrolysis

➤ **What It Is:** This method removes hair permanently with electric current.

➤ **How It Works:** A trained technician inserts a needle or probe into the hair follicle and passes an electric current, which is converted into heat, through the follicle. Each hair is treated individually, so the process may take several sessions. Minor skin trauma—dark spots and scarring—can be a side effect of electrolysis, so it is important that you find a technician who is experienced working with darker skin tones. Sessions cost between $15 and $100.

➤ **Best Use:** Electrolysis removes hair from your face, underarms, arms, stomach and bikini area.

Lasers

➤ **What It Is:** Although this method doesn't get rid of hair permanently, the results can last for months; and when hair returns, it may be thinner.

➤ **How It Works:** Lasers emit a light that destroys hair follicles. The best type for Black skins use longer wavelengths to focus on hair follicles without damaging the skin. Laser removal may require several sessions. Sessions can run from $150 and up.

➤ **Best Use:** Face, underarms, arms, stomach and bikini area may all be lasered for hair removal.

Intense Pulse Light (IPL)

➤ **What It Is:** IPL is a nonpermanent laserlike hair removal technique.

➤ **How It Works:** Multiple wavelengths of light beam into follicles to destroy hair. Although this method significantly reduces hair growth after repeated treatments, it is unsafe for people of color unless used with a specific filter (known as a 755 filter) that allows for greater pauses between light pulses. Without this cooling time, IPL could be seriously damaging to Black skin. This technique should be administered by a professional who is experienced in working with people of color. Sessions cost from $150 to $3,000.

➤ **Best Use:** IPL is used on the face, underarms, arms, stomach and bikini area.

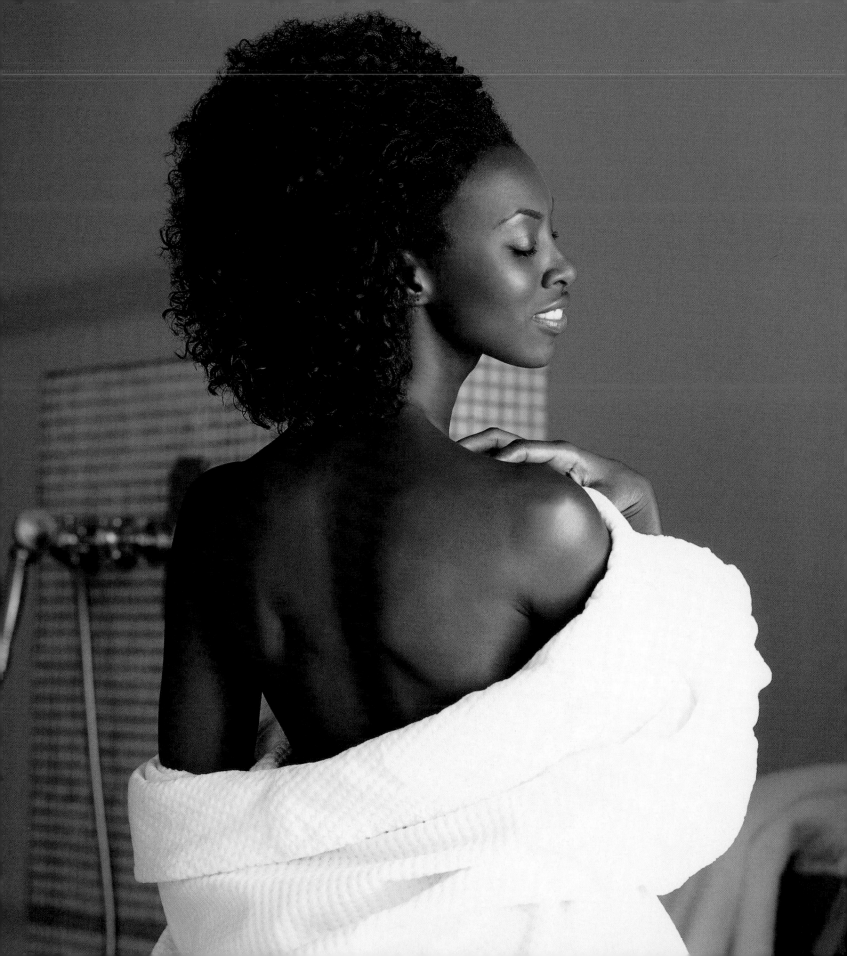

Prepare to Pamper

No matter how hectic life may seem, you must take the time to recharge, regroup and do something just for you. Body work, including aromatherapy and healing massage, can help you relax and promote beauty both inside and out. So when you can, carve out time to treat yourself to these bodywork treatments designed to leave you refreshed, renewed and rejuvenated.

Aromatherapy

What It Is: Aromatherapy uses a variety of scented essential oils to help heal and relax the body by stimulating the olfactory senses and the brain.

How It Works: Tailor your selections to your wellness needs. Need to feel invigorated? Try some eucalyptus. Want to calm down? Lather on lavender. Other aromatic blends can help to soothe if you are suffering from headaches, digestive problems or even PMS. Oils can also be added to classic spa treatments like facials, manicures and pedicures. And although aromatherapy is not usually considered dangerous, certain oils (sage, peppermint, cedar wood) can have an adverse effect on fetuses, so pregnant women should consult their doctor before booking any appointments.

Soothing Scents

Essential oils add healing benefits to bath and body treatments. Mix and match oils based on your scent preference and wellness needs. Base oils like jojoba and almond complement all others.

Oil	Best For
Grapefruit	Boosting energy
Marjoram	Enhancing circulation
Eucalyptus	Easing tightness and cooling
Peppermint	Elevating mood
Birch	Easing tightness
Lavender	Calming and healing
Chamomile	Calming
Rose	Battling insomnia and PMS
Wintergreen	Stimulating and cooling
Clary sage	Soothing and relaxing
Lemon	Soothing and relaxing
Jasmine	Invigorating
Rosemary	Boosting energy and mental stimulation; clearing congestion

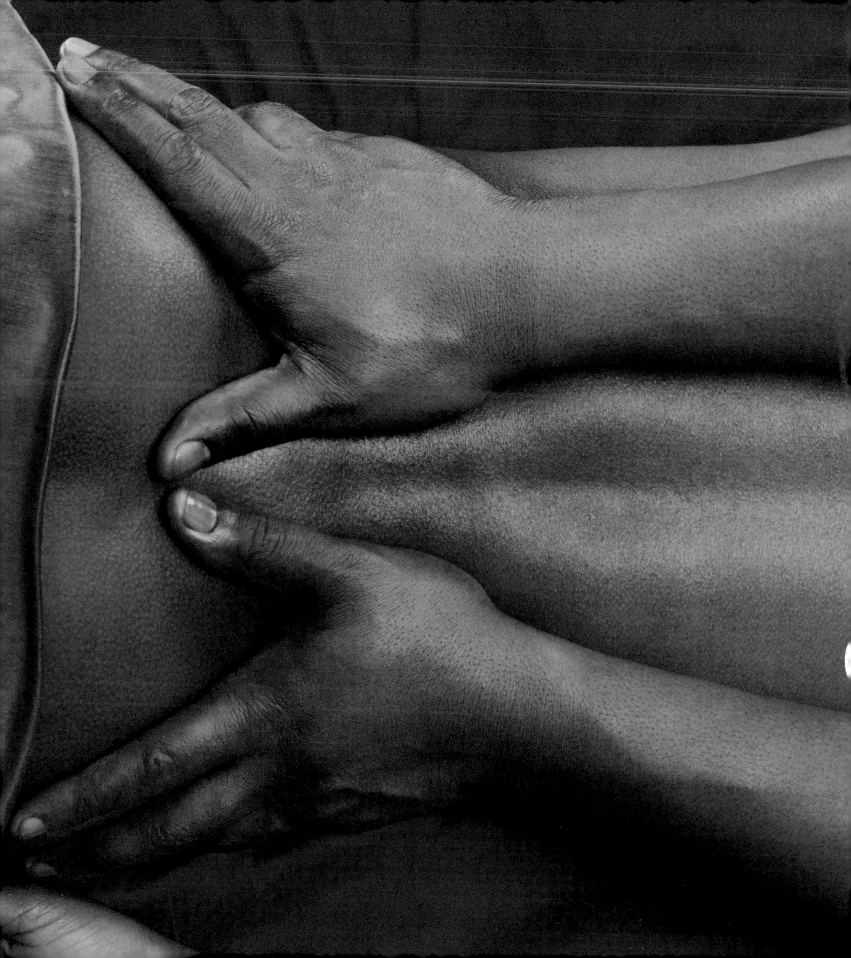

Massage

Massage is the manipulation of body tissues by rubbing, kneading or tapping with hands or instruments, which causes knotted muscles to relax and helps heal the body. It is based on the idea that our bodies are one continuous flow of energy. Different techniques—including kneading, pulling and stroking—are said to increase circulation, relieve muscle pain and stiffness, reduce blood pressure, improve flexibility and strengthen the immune system. You can choose from many different types of massage, some of which are described here.

Swedish

What It Is: Swedish is the most basic of all massages, using long smooth strokes, kneading movements, circular pressure, and tapping and scratching with the fingers.

How It Works: Swedish massage increases the flow of oxygenated blood to tight muscle tissues. This helps release toxins from the tissues and organs and relieve stress.

Best Use: Most healthy individuals can benefit from a Swedish massage, especially if they receive one every three to six months.

Deep-Tissue

What It Is: Deep-tissue massage is done through the use of slow hand strokes and deep finger pressure.

How It Works: This massage reaches the deeper layers of muscle tissue by warming up tightened areas to release chronic tension in the body. Although you may experience some soreness afterward, it is only temporary.

Best Use: Deep-tissue techniques have many benefits. Ideally, they help those with muscular and skeletal problems such as tendonitis, torn muscles, sprains and some forms of bursitis, making it great for athletes. This massage also helps alleviate neck and lower-back pain.

Hot Stone

What It Is: This treatment uses heated volcanic stones (135° to 150°).

How It Works: The massage therapist places additional stones along the spine over the seven chakras (a Sanskrit term for the major energy centers situated along the spine). The stones may also be placed in the hands, between toes and beneath shoulders.

Best Use: Hot stones are great for those suffering from sore muscles or other aches and pains, since the heat from the stones penetrates the body three times more deeply than heat generated from hands. This method may not be suitable for everyone, especially pregnant women and those with diabetes. If one of these conditions applies to you, make sure to consult a physician before indulging.

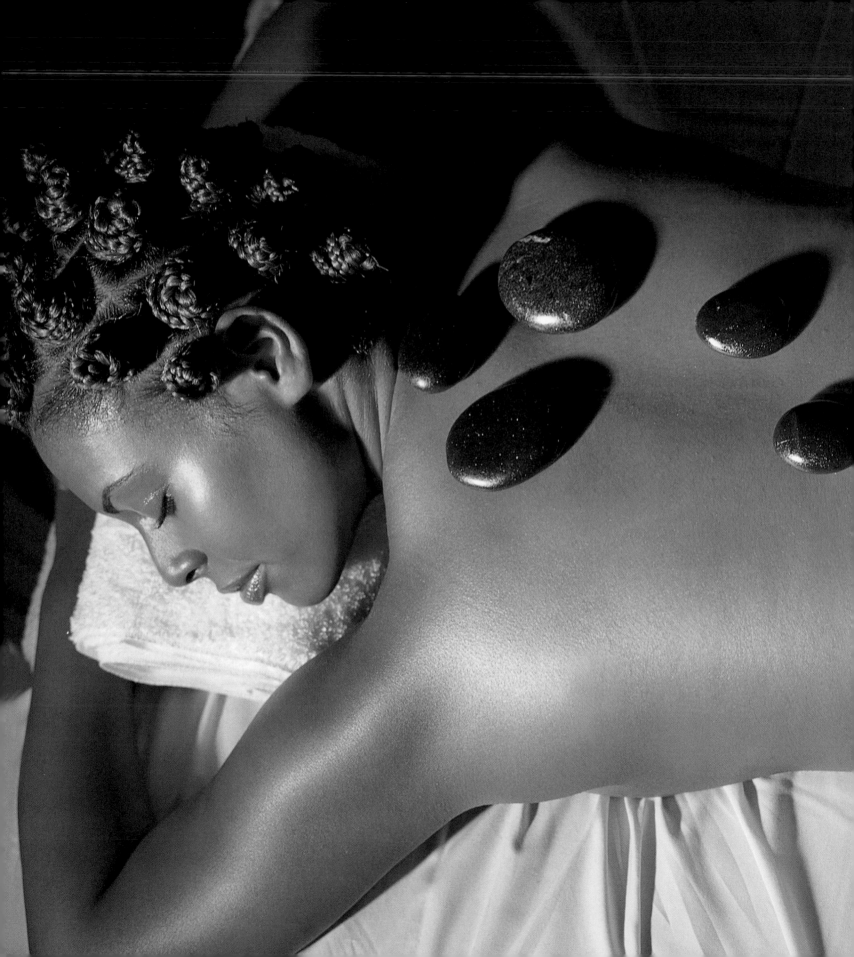

Drink a glass of freshly juiced celery, apple and carrots to help break down the fat cells that form cellulite.

Throw a Spa Party

For a great way to get pampered and socialize at the same time, organize a group of sisterfriends for a spa day. Pick a day spa and negotiate a group deal. Or try an at-home pampering session. Several day spas offer mobile services, where trained professionals bring the pampering to you. You can also look for one of the many do-it-yourself kits sold in stores that contain all the goodies needed for an at-home spa party. Friends can take turns giving and receiving manicures, pedicures and facial masks, while sitting back and enjoying each other's company.

4 Home Spa Essentials

➤ **Scented candles:** Choose scents with aromatherapy benefits, ones that promise to illuminate for hours or decorous styles adorned with pressed flowers or dried fruit.
➤ **A foot soak:** To revive tired tootsies, try mineral salts.
➤ **A facial mask:** Take advantage of your time in the tub by multitasking: Apply a deep-cleaning mask to your face while you soak.
➤ **A bath treat:** Taking a long, luxurious body soak is a wonderful way to fully immerse yourself in the spa experience.

At-Home Spa Care

Sometimes, as much as we want to get away, going to the spa for a quick getaway is just not in the budget. But that obstacle shouldn't prevent you from making me-time. You can easily pamper yourself by creating an at-home spa tailored to your needs. All you need is the willingness to free yourself from the cares of the world, a few products and some precious hours, and the pampering can begin. Here are four ways to get your home spa ready for relaxation.

Stock up on spa accessories. Buy items like scented candles, specialty soaks, bath treats, moisturizers and massage oils to re-create the spa experience at home.

Build your own sanctuary. With a little imagination and the right touches, your home can easily assume a soothing spalike atmosphere. Try dimming the lights, burning aromatherapy candles or oil lamps and playing relaxing music for a calming ambiance.

Remove unnecessary clutter. Just keep the staples like body and face towels, bowls for facials and manicures and a large basin for foot soaks.

Free yourself from distractions. Turn off telephones and pagers. This unselfish gesture will help you relax and release you from your responsibilities and distractions.

Photography Credits